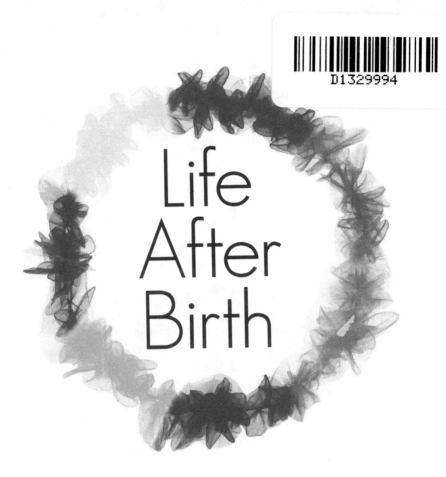

Life After Birth

A Parent's Holistic Guide for Thriving in the Fourth Trimester

DIANE S. SPEIER

Praeclarus Press, LLC
www.PraeclarusPress.com

Praeclarus Press, LLC
2504 Sweetgum Lane
Amarillo, Texas 79124 USA
806-367-9950
www.PraeclarusPress.com

DISCLAIMER

The information contained in this publication is advisory only and is not intended to replace sound clinical judgment or individualized patient care. The author disclaims all warranties, whether expressed or implied, including any warranty as the quality, accuracy, safety, or suitability of this information for any particular purpose.

ISBN: 978-1-946665-22-5

Cover Design: Ken Tackett
Developmental Editing: Kathleen Kendall-Tackett
Copyediting: Chris Tackett
Layout & Design: Nelly Murariu

Dedication

To Jasper and Olivia,

and
future generations of parents
who value practical and holistic ways
to thrive in the fourth trimester
while making the transition to parenthood.

Acknowledgements

The process of writing of this book began more than six years ago, but was percolating in my mind for much longer. As a birth professional, I noticed there have been so few books written that focused on the time right after birth, (there were only a handful that I was aware of that had been written on the subject over 40 years), and many that are written end up concentrating on what goes wrong, such as perinatal mood and anxiety disorders. Although it's important to bring awareness to something that disrupts the lives of up to 20% of women after birth, what about the other 80% who are well and still need information and support as they navigate the transition to parenthood?

One of the inspirations for this book came from my daughter, Mariel Sands, who asked me after the birth of her first child, "Where are all the books on the postpartum period?" I remember that conversation in the car as we were driving back from an appointment with the pediatrician soon after my grandson was born. It prompted me to start writing, drawing on many years of experience and expertise working with postpartum women. Mariel used to come with me (when she was little) as I taught my mother and baby exercise classes, and I think she had an expectation that there would be lots of information about this transitional time. I am grateful for the conversation that got the ball rolling.

A book like this couldn't have been written if I hadn't had children of my own. That experience inspired me to become a birth professional and postpartum specialist, working with families in California, New York and the north west of England. My youngest son, Jasper, and his partner Olivia, were my "millennial" consultants, who advised me on what their generation resonates with and how to appeal to them with their own personal perspectives. Raising a family is on the job training, and my family were the stimulus for many career decisions that I've made that have culminated in this book.

Another thank you goes to Emma Dillon, who is the lovely model for the energy medicine techniques that are disseminated throughout the book. I couldn't have found a better person to demonstrate the various postures, and help the reader understand how to do the practices that augment self-care in the fourth trimester. Thank you, Emma, for your lightness of being. Kudos to Gary Dillon, whose professional photography skills put the finishing touches on the photos that show how the techniques look. Thank you for the hours you devoted to making those photos picture perfect!

Donna Eden is an inspiring pioneer in energy medicine and the founder of Eden Energy Medicine. When I read Eden's book on *Energy Medicine for Women,* I noticed that ironically there was very little in the way of information about pregnancy, birth, and the postpartum period. While I was training in EEM, Donna and I had a conversation with David Feinstein about my interest in applying EEM to the postpartum period, and they were enthusiastic and supportive of my efforts to fill the gap. I hope this book measures up. I am grateful for permission to reproduce two Innersource (the EEM organization) diagrams that have been included in the energy medicine chapters. To learn more about Donna Eden and Eden Energy Medicine go to: www.LearnEnergyMedicine.com

My friend and colleague, Elly Taylor, has been a great support over the years as the book progressed. As often happens these days, Elly and I met on Facebook and we learned we had a lot of common ground in our focus on what happens after birth. Our collaboration on a couple of conference presentations is something that can only have happened with the advent of global technology in the 21st century, being that Elly lives in Australia and I live in the UK. Elly read an early draft of this book, when it became the postnatal app, *Digital Doula*' (the app supports and complements this book). It is remarkable that we've only actually met in person twice in all these years; yet this relationship has been a blessing. Elly also put her two cents in when the title of the book was going through various permutations, and reminded me that the important idea was life after birth. Thank you for your friendship, support, and inspiration.

Phyllis Klaus, who generously agreed to write the foreword to this book, has been a friend and colleague for 35 years. We met at a Pre and Perinatal Psychology Association of North America (PPPANA) conference in 1983 and found we had many shared interests around birth and beyond. We would meet up at each biennial Congress (PPPANA became APPPAH, Association for Prenatal and Perinatal Psychology and Health) and would indulge in lengthy conversations about the postpartum period.

Those conversations were instrumental in my original ideas for writing a book on the postpartum period. I am so grateful for Phyllis's friendship and support over the years, even when we saw less of each other when I moved to the UK. Thank you, Phyl, for all that you are, and all that you give.

To those who agreed to review this book early on, I appreciate the time and effort involved in taking on a project like this, and I am deeply grateful that you have been willing to make it happen: Vicki Matthews, Francoise Freedman, Michel Odent, Robin Lim, and Jack Travis.

I am grateful for the help Vanessa McInerney Vanderhoek provided regarding information and links on maternity and parental leave policy in Australia, and to Emma Catteau who helped me access leave information in France.

I am blessed with two very special friends, Elena Karplus and Sonia Still, who have been cheering me on from afar through conversations, social media, and the wonderful access that phone apps offer! The loving friendship and support through life's various vicissitudes, and different time zones, has meant more than you can imagine.

Over the years, my clients have been enthusiastic participants in groups, classes, workshops and doula care, helping me to fine tune the message for what parents need during the childbearing year. The privilege of being there when babies are born, or when mothers need help after birth, and educating parents in how they can meet the challenges of birth and the fourth trimester, has been a delightful and heartfelt experience for me for decades.

Kathleen Kendall-Tackett, my publisher and editor-in-chief, succeeded in restructuring the book in a way that has vastly improved it, while keeping the essential content that I wrote. It is thrilling to see how the collaboration worked, as we journeyed through the editing process together. Some personal health matters meant things went more slowly than anticipated, and I thank you for your patience and perseverance. I am also grateful that you recognized that the last "chapter" that I was writing had actually grown into another book that will be published soon after this one. Thanks to Ken Tackett, who steered the book through production and created the cover, and Nelly Murariu, who wonderfully shaped this book into its present form.

As mentioned above, Shannon Hicks has redeveloped the postnatal app that complements this book, *Digital Doula*', which is available on a cross-platform basis for iOS and Android: http://digitaldoula.com/. The app includes supplemental information on a number of subjects related to the content of this book, including access to the links that are included throughout the book.

And finally, Margaret Brade, my life-partner who has kept me afloat through the years, and who understood the importance of getting the book written! In conversations about our future, she would remind me to get the book done so the world could benefit. Thank you for your love, and for holding the vision with me for the publication of this book, and much more.

Foreword

by Phyllis Klaus LMFT, LMSW

Life After Birth: A Parent's Holistic Guide for Thriving in the Fourth Trimester

Diane Speier has written a book I wish had been available when I had my three children many years ago. This is a book whose time has come; actually, has been overdue! I consider her knowledge, her experience, and her research presented with clarity, skill, and compassion as essential information for every woman expecting a baby. I feel privileged to write this foreword. I have known Dr. Speier for about 35 years and have admired her superb programs dealing with the needs of women during pregnancy, birth, and the postpartum period. She has the expertise of not only having lived the experience of parenting herself but has created hundreds of programs for other mothers and families, and researched this period of life for her PhD, developing a deep understanding. This book has incorporated a whole new level of information made palatable, easily taken in, digested, and available to new birthing families.

My own involvement in birth was inspired by working with my husband Dr. Marshall Klaus and our colleague Dr. John Kennell in bringing the bonding and doula studies to families. These elements have become fundamental to helping families. As I became immersed in the perinatal experience, I recognized the unmet needs of the postpartum family. Interestingly, the first lecture I presented I called "The Postpartum Period: The Neglected Phase of Childbirth."

Diane's own work is inspirational. She was among the first to recognize that women needed other women, and created groups for new mothers focusing on the adjustment to new parenting. Helping women regain their health and strength, she formed postpartum exercise classes. She supported women in processing their emotions and in enhancing their relationships. In this book, she has carefully described the importance of partner communication and the sensitivity of new roles and needs. She recognizes how important help for breastfeeding is and how to strengthen bonding and attachment.

She decodes the effect of hormones during and after the birth process. She describes complex physiological changes in a very easy to understand manner in her section on hormones. She explains in thoughtful detail how to take care of one's body after birth as a very personal, intimate dimension to enable healing.

She has introduced a subject that has not always been available to modern audiences, which is Energy Medicine. She has described and presented exercises that are tapping into an energetic level of the body. It is an ancient method that has been redefined in modern terms to recreate balance physically and emotionally. She describes beautifully the Eden Energy Medicine Method and how these movements and actions can do much to create healing in the body, mind and spirit.

The language of this book is personal; it speaks directly to you, and she explains the meaning of words and conditions that professionals use in relatable ways that are easy to remember. She has created a work that brings this essential healing information and resources to parents in an accessible and understandable manner.

She has a very deep level of knowledge about all of these processes. She has very excellent resources and other methods that she interweaves into her own work, which has enriched every dimension of this period of personal growth and change. This book is to be read slowly and savored. I encourage readers to follow some of the methods she presents for emotional, physical, and interpersonal development and strength during the richness of this pivotal period of life.

►◄

Phyllis Klaus LMFT, LMSW is a psychotherapist working with families in the perinatal period for over 40 years. She co-authored *Your Amazing Newborn, Bonding, The Doula Book,* and *When Survivors Give Birth.* She is a founder of DONA International and PATTCh (Prevention and Treatment of Traumatic Childbirth).

Contents

Introduction

Congratulations! You've either just had a baby, or you will be having one soon. Ideally, this book is designed to be read while you are still pregnant because it will help you to prepare for what's to come, allowing you to implement some of the ideas before the baby comes. However, I expect most of my readers will have already had their babies, so whether it's before or after birth, you can implement those perspectives that resonate with you.

I have been a birth professional for 40 years, and want to help new mothers make the best transition to parenthood possible, through groups, classes, the research I've done, and individual counseling. With all the books that are written about pregnancy, birth, and parenting, why are there such limited resources about the postpartum period? Most postpartum books focus on what goes wrong during this pivotal time, and there are only a handful of books that dwell on what's positive and possible in the transition to parenthood. I hope that I can fill this gap with practical and useful information that you can draw on as you step onto the path of new motherhood. Through you, I hope to help your partner to be present for you in a supportive role, and to enrich the experience of fatherhood/parenthood, honoring the importance of the partner's involvement in the development of the baby, and fostering the connection between you as your relationship is redefined and expanded by your lives as parents. In this introduction, I share with you my own journey in facilitating women becoming mothers through the years.

The name of this book was originally *Handbook for the Postnatal Period*, and reflected the influence of the UK, where I live. "After birth" is called postnatal, which is the precise meaning: post – after, natal – birth. Once the manuscript was submitted to the publisher, all the "postnatals" were converted into "postpartums," which is the term used in the U.S. Over the course of the editing process, the name of the book went through several permutations, and at one time it was *A User's Guide to the Postpartum*

Period. The Brits objected to the use of postpartum, which is not a common term here, so we gave it some more consideration. We decided the focus could be on the fourth trimester, that bypassed either postnatal or postpartum. We wanted to focus on life after birth, and through a poll on Facebook, the consensus was *Life After Birth: A Parent's Holistic Guide for Thriving in the Fourth Trimester.* This title says exactly what's in the tin!

My Journey

Postpartum Support Groups

My interest in the postpartum period began when I became a certified childbirth educator back in 1978. With my background in psychology, I always felt curious about how women adjust to becoming mothers from a psychological perspective, and this led me to create a postpartum support group. I called it *And Baby Makes 3.* This was a group for new mothers who came together to share their experiences, both positive and negative, and to learn from each other. An unspoken aspect of this group experience was the sense of community it created, bringing women who were at the same stage in life into a supportive network with each other. In those days, networking happened on a face-to-face basis!

On a personal level, I had two young children at the time, and after the birth of my second son, I experienced a subclinical case of postpartum depression: not enough to disable me, but enough to not feel right for a number of months. If there had been a group where I could have expressed my feelings, I think it would have been a healing framework to work through the issues I was having. It was when I joined a women's group (the consciousness-raising kind of that era) that I realized that I had been suffering a mild depression, and the support of other women was instrumental in returning me to my normal self.

Another inspiration for this group was a book that had just been published called *Mothercare*, by Lyn DelliQuadri and Kati Breckenridge, which advocated for supporting women through this important transition into parenthood. Posting flyers on notice boards attracted the attention of a talk radio reporter, who interviewed me about the group I was developing.

Lyn DelliQuadri contacted me at this time, when she was producing a video based on her book, and she was looking for potential "actors" to film. In principle I liked the idea, but the practical reality of a film crew in the home at this vulnerable time in a woman's life was not popular. I didn't recruit for her film, and we lost touch, so I don't know what happened with it. But I felt even more resolved about the importance of supporting mothers through this time.

After our family moved back to New York in 1980, I was soon pregnant with my daughter, and was learning the lay of the land as both a pregnant woman and a childbirth educator. I was networking with maternity care providers, childbirth educators, and mothers to get a sense of the resources that were available to women/mothers at that time. Planning a homebirth connected me with the underground movement of alternative birth choices in order to locate a homebirth midwife in the area. After starting with midwives who worked and lived in New York City, when we lived in the northern suburbs (and one of them did not drive), I decided to change midwives. The choice was based on a new friend's experience of having to send someone to collect the midwife when she went into labor. I knew that wouldn't work for me.

Since homebirth midwives were few and far between in those days, I ended up with a midwife who worked in an adjacent county and lived in northern New Jersey. I found out about her from women at a La Leche League meeting that I had been attending. La Leche League International (LLLI) is the grassroots organization that was created in the late 1950s by women who were looking for information and support while breastfeeding, and has grown into an international presence around the world for all kinds of breastfeeding knowledge and expert advice. Although many women, like me, attended meetings before birth, most were new mothers going through the trials and tribulations of the postpartum period, and were benefiting by the breastfeeding support. It was one of the few postpartum group experiences that was available at the time.

I had attended League meetings both in California and New York and was troubled by some of their beliefs, particularly around returning to work. There were positive stories of mothers who had gone back to work and successfully continued to breastfeed. I was surprised that their success was not recognized in a positive way. I wanted to provide a different type

type of group experience for new mothers. Since then, La Leche League has evolved, and has published several books acknowledging women who work and want to continue to breastfeed. It was a long time coming, but at the time, it was the reason that I stopped attending meetings. I would like to acknowledge, however, that the information that LLLI provides on the subject is excellent, and the breastfeeding support that they offer by telephone for struggling mothers is second to none.

Postpartum Exercise Classes

After my daughter was born, I was looking for something to do with her while my sons were at school. I ran a couple of groups and found that what mothers were most concerned about was getting back into shape and finding something they could do with their babies, and *Reshape and Unwind* was born. This was a postpartum exercise class for mothers and babies that included infant exercise and baby massage instruction. I attended classes like this when my sons were little in New York City with Suzy Prudden, the only person I knew that taught mother and baby classes, and I modeled my classes on her work. Suzy was a fitness guru at the time, and an exercise inspiration for me. In the last year of living in California (we lived there from 1977 to 1980), I had been a regular attendee of Jane Fonda's Workout in Beverly Hills, and had become a fitness enthusiast, which gave momentum to my decision to create an exercise class for mothers and babies.

Another model that I used was the format set up by Femmy Delyser, who created the program for pregnant and postpartum women at Jane Fonda's Workout, and who I knew as a childbirth educator colleague. Suzy inspired the activities for babies, and Femmy inspired the mothers' workout that I created to help them get back into shape. It was a synthesis of both with a focus on both mother and baby. It ran for 20 years and finished after I emigrated to the UK and ran the class through a local leisure center, and then independently for a while.

A by-product of these classes was the community that was created for mothers who continued to meet with each other long after they finished the course with me. I would bump into women in the community who told me that they were still friends with women they had met in my classes 10 years before. And their children were friends too! When I was promoting these classes to the local pediatricians, the sympathetic comments they made acknowledged how these classes would provide the kind of experience that women living in cities would find at the park bench. Women of the suburbs often felt isolated in their homes, not having a place to gather with other mothers, and what I was doing was filling a gap. The doctors supported my efforts, and the classes were popular with mothers.

The benefit for me was my own personal fitness over 20 years. I listened to mothers' concerns, and provided an oasis for new mothers to express their deepest issues and share their wisdom with others in a beautiful exchange of caring support for each other. That is truly the essence of community, and I am delighted that I have contributed to that by facilitating these offerings for new mothers in various locations.

I also worked over the years as a doula, the Greek word for servant, who mothers the mother during labor and the postpartum period. Being a birth doula was something I had done with my clients going back to 1978, and I attended births in California and New York in birth centers and hospitals. Channeling birth energy was something that I was particularly good at. I also functioned as a postpartum doula, going into the home and doing various household tasks that would allow the mother to focus her attention on the baby and the relationship that was developing between her and her newborn.

In 1995, I created a doula service for birth and the postpartum period. The majority of my clients were women who were childbirth preparation students, but I was also listed in various resources for doula care in which I worked with women who did not know me in that context. Many of my postpartum doula clients started as strangers, but I loved serving women in that capacity, and we bonded in the days when I was visiting them in their homes. It was great to be able to open a space for them to integrate their new baby into their lives in a healthy and positive way.

Continued Professional Development

While I was teaching *Reshape and Unwind*, I went back to graduate school to get my Master's Degree in Applied Psychology, with a specialty in The Psychology of Parenthood. Working with mothers over the years had inspired me to take it to a new level in studying the subject within an academic context. When I conducted research into new motherhood, I was able to use the classes as a source of participants and as a context for studying mothers. The everyday experience of working with mothers and studying parenthood dovetailed nicely, culminating in an MA in 1994. I loved watching women mature into motherhood, connected to their babies and others through the context of an exercise class.

My studies enriched my awareness of the transition to parenthood from an intellectual perspective, which were translated into my interactions with my clients. As I grew in knowledge and wisdom, I shared this with women, always striving to provide the best experience that would facilitate this transition for them, with a specific focus on the early months after giving birth. My expertise was grounded in my work with mothers and the education/training that provided the theory that informed that work.

When I emigrated to the UK in 1998, I again became a postgraduate student studying for my PhD in Women's Studies. The feminist research that I conducted used my case notes as a certified childbirth educator as the data for analysis in my thesis (*The Childbirth Educator as Ethnographer: A Feminist Retrospective Ethnography of a Professional Practice*, University of Manchester, 2002). The reflective reading that informed my thesis uncovered certain themes in the accounts of birth that my birth clients had told me over the 10 years that were the focus of this research. They were knowledge, support, and empowerment, or knowledge + support = empowerment. The research strengthened my feminist awareness, and I applied it to the work that I had done with both pregnant and postpartum women over the years. I was looking at the transition to parenthood with a feminist lens, and noticing the gap in feminism when it came to birth and becoming a mother. I published an article called "Becoming a Mother" in the *Journal for the Association for Research on Mothering* (ARM) in 2001. The article concentrated on the number of choices women make on the journey to becoming mothers in a society where mothering seems to be an imperative role for women. The feminist focus on reproductive rights was more about if and when to have children, and the attitude towards mothering was constrained due to the emphasis on women's place in the marketplace. Childbirth was far too biologically deterministic for feminists to embrace during the Third Wave. That birth could be an empowering experience, particularly with knowledge and support, was my contribution to the literature.

My first job as an academic researcher was on a randomized controlled trial (RCT, the so-called gold standard for health research) on postpartum depression. In the UK, there is a nursing specialty called a health visitor, who does additional training for this position, and whose role as a public health nurse is to facilitate the transition to parenthood by visiting the mother in her home for a number of weeks after the midwife signs off. I was a local research coordinator working with health visitors attached to general practices in the study comparing the effectiveness of different counseling approaches to postpartum depression. Health visitors were trained in either person-centered counseling or cognitive-behavioral counseling before the onset of the study, and they counseled women who had postpartum depression using one of these techniques. They used the Edinburgh Postnatal Depression Scale (EPDS) to measure postpartum depression, and those women in the study who scored above the threshold were offered counseling. I traveled around the area visiting health visitors and helping to recruit participants for a year and a half and then started on another study on postpartum health, which I did concurrently for another nine months.

This postpartum health study developed a survey that would measure postpartum health and wellbeing, and I was happy to be working on something positive around new parenthood. So much theory about the transition is based on pathology in the same way that health is sometimes defined as the absence of disease. I was the qualitative researcher on this project and interviewed 52 participants, both mothers and fathers, to get a sense of what their experience was like in the weeks and months following their babies' births. What were the challenges and what were the healthy aspects of this period in their lives? The analysis of the data generated items for the *Sheffield Postnatal Health Instrument*, which was mailed to more than 1,000 women and their partners, and measured various elements of life in the early days. My contract on this study finished before the final instrument was fine-tuned, and the first article to come out of the research was published in 2011 in the *Quality of Life Research Journal*.

My career as a health researcher took me further and further away from birth and the postpartum period with the next projects that I worked on, and after seven years of academic research, I decided to return to the work I felt passionately about: birth and the postpartum period. When my last contract ended, I left academia to become self-employed again as a birth professional. I resumed the provision of doula care and became a recognized birth and postpartum doula in the UK after taking a training course and being fast-tracked through the recognition process with Doula UK. An inspiration for this return to the work I love was the birth of my step-granddaughter in 2009. I taught birth preparation classes to her parents and was the doula during her birth, which reawakened the impulse to engage with families again at this precious moment in life.

In 2011, my daughter gave birth to my grandson in Los Angeles, and I was able to be with her when he was six days old for a couple of weeks, and again for another couple of weeks the following month. Being a doula for my grandchild was wonderful (my granddaughter was born in 2005, and I also spent a few days with her in the early weeks), and my connection with my daughter blossomed too. Her experience of the postpartum period gave momentum to the decision to write this book, and we've been able to incorporate her perceptions and struggles into the content of this book. She was the co-creator of the app for this book, *Digital Doula*', and we collaborated on this project for the benefit of new mothers everywhere.

Is There Life after Birth?

I've often laughed with parents over this question because when they were preparing for childbirth, they really could not see beyond the birth process. Nothing about the time after birth penetrates because the birth looms so large. Then they felt lost once the birth was over because they didn't process the information that I gave them about the postpartum period, breastfeeding, or babycare. When I restructured my Birth Empowerment Childbirth Preparation' classes, I made the first class a Saturday workshop for women only about staying healthy during pregnancy, four classes on labor and delivery for couples, and then a Sunday seminar for couples about what happens after the baby is born. It was a chance to get hands-on experience of changing a diaper/nappy and baby clothes on a (Cabbage Patch!) doll and learn about other postpartum matters. Even before the structural change, I encouraged people to take notes so they could refer to them later when needed. In one class, I had a couple of pregnant obstetricians as clients, who took copious notes about breastfeeding and other new-parenting information that was not part of their knowledge base.

For this reason, *Life After Birth: A Parent's Holistic Guide for Thriving in the Fourth Trimester* has been written to accommodate this tendency not to hear anything about what happens after the birth. It can be taken to the birthplace for ready reference immediately after birth. It can be used thereafter as something to reference on a particular subject or to be read through to get an overall sense of what this singular time in life is all about. It is designed to provide strategies for managing the intensity of change that is taking place and increasing your understanding of the dramatic fluctuations that occur with your hormones, your moods, and your energy levels. Knowledge is power, and I hope that you will feel empowered by the suggestions made to help you make the most of this transition because ultimately you will come to realize that *you* are the expert of your own life and your baby. I would like to help you rely less on "experts" (even though I am one!), and tune in to your latent intuition, and the information that is contained in this book is geared for that unfolding.

ACOG Committee Opinion on Postpartum Care

Speaking of experts, in May 2018, while this book was in the editing stage, the American College of Obstetricians and Gynecologists (ACOG) issued a Committee Opinion that redefined the Postpartum Visit after birth. #736 (2018) replaced #666 (2016), drawing on the expertise of the Academy of Breastfeeding Medicine, the American College of Nurse-Midwives, the National Association of Nurse Practitioners in Women's Health, the Society for Academic Specialists in General Obstetrics and Gynecology, and the Society for Maternal-Fetal Medicine. The Committee Opinion was developed by the ACOG Presidential Task Force on Redefining the Postpartum Visit and the Committee on Obstetric Practice. It's called "Optimizing Postpartum Care," and provides recommendations and conclusions for a new pattern of postpartum care from medical providers.

The American system for postpartum care has always been a visit to the obstetrician between 4 to 6 weeks after delivery, although with midwives the pattern is different. As more than 98% of births take place in hospitals (Doyle, n.d.) (https://www.scientificamerican.com/article/out-of-hospital-births-on-the-rise-in-u-s/), and just over 8% of American births are attended by midwives in the U.S. (ACNM, 2016) (http://www.midwife.org/CNM/CM-attended-Birth-Statistics), postpartum care is overwhelmingly managed by obstetric practice. By comparison, in the UK, where midwives are the first point of contact during pregnancy, midwives did over 75% of deliveries in 1989-1990. This rate has steadily declined over the years to just 53% in 2015 to 2016, reflecting the increased medicalization of the perinatal period in the UK (Stephenson, 2016) (https://www.nursingtimes.net/news/hospital/only-half-of-babies-in-england-now-delivered-by-midwives/7013310.article). This upgrade to the American provision of postpartum care is significant, with the biggest change being that now mothers will be seen within the first three weeks after birth, rather than the common six-week visit. So much can go wrong in those first six weeks, especially for the mental health of the mother and her family.

This new paradigm for postpartum care reinforces the importance of the fourth trimester in which women recover from birth and nurture their infants. Rather than a single visit to the doctor, postpartum care is now reconceptualized as an ongoing process that sets the stage for long-term health and wellbeing. An initial assessment is done within the first *three* weeks postpartum, followed up with ongoing care as needed, and concluding with a comprehensive visit no later than 12 weeks postpartum. The comprehensive visit should include a full assessment of physical, social, and psychological wellbeing, covering the following areas: mood and emotional wellbeing; infant care and feeding; sexuality, contraception and birth spacing; sleep and fatigue; physical recovery from birth; chronic disease management; and health maintenance. One health care provider would be assigned as the care coordinator for any ongoing care in the primary-care domain. Optimizing care and support would require policy changes, including insurance reimbursement policies that acknowledge the ongoing process of postpartum care instead of a one-time visit.

One valuable aspect of the new paradigm is the development of a post-partum care plan addressing the transition to parenthood and well-woman care. You will find in the first part of this book, The Fourth Trimester, a Postpartum W.E.L.L.N.E.S.S. Plan that was devised to help you thrive during the stressful transition that is happening. I was excited to learn that ACOG, who has rarely been on the forefront of progress in maternity care, has established the importance of a postpartum plan for families inclusive of medical provision. The comprehensive visit would be individualized and woman-centered. In addition to the woman and her obstetric team, the "care team" includes family and friends, providing social and material support, as well as medical providers responsible for the clinical care of the mother and her infant. When the plan is initiated during the prenatal period, anticipatory guidance can be woven within it, and just 15 minutes of anticipatory guidance is known to improve maternal well-being (with less depression and breastfeeding problems). The postpartum plan would be reviewed and updated after the birth occurs, to reflect any potential trauma or other adverse or unexpected outcomes of the birth (ACOG, 2018).

Up to 40% of women don't attend a postpartum visit, and the new Opinion statement seeks to increase the level of engagement with patients after birth. It also owns up to the reality that "for many women in the United States, the 6-week postpartum visit punctuates a period *devoid of formal or informal maternal support*" (emphasis mine; ACOG, 2018, p. e141). This book addresses that void of support, though it does not claim to be offering medical advice to its readers. If you feel that something is wrong with your health, please see a medical provider if this new intention of ACOG has not been implemented with a real plan for your medical care. The causes of maternal morbidity (illness) can occur during the first 10 days after birth, and over half of pregnancy-related maternal deaths occur after birth. Seeing the doctor can protect you and your infant from these devastating situations, and the new paradigm includes essential follow-up for women at high risk of complications. Please don't hesitate.

It's not clear how long it will take to implement this new paradigm for postpartum care. It could be that some obstetrician/gynecologists enthusiastically adopt this comprehensive course of action, while others resist the changes it would require. Midwives already practice many of the components of supportive care for their patients. Obstetrics is now making

Energy Medicine to the Rescue

Energy medicine is a system of healing that works on the premise that energy is a living, moving force that defines our state of health and happiness. Using energy medicine for self-care, you can activate your body's natural healing abilities in a way that restores flow, balance, and harmony to your life. The energy medicine that I use in this book comes from Eden Energy Medicine, drawing on the work of Donna Eden, a pioneer in the field. Her book, *Energy Medicine* (1998), is a classic and well worth reading. There are energy-healing practices at the end of each Part that can help you to manage your experience. The Daily Energy Routine in Part One is a wonderful way to work with your energy through a 10-minute set of movements that restores your balance and energy flow. Ten minutes might feel like an eternity during the postpartum period, but the investment will reap dividends, and you can always do some of it if you cannot do the whole routine.

The energy-medicine tools for Part Two are designed to calm and balance you as you travel along the hormonal roller coaster of postpartum life. By working with the meridians (energy pathways) that govern the stress response, along with other energy points that stabilize and promote healing, you can restore your center of gravity while things whirl around you. In Part Three, there are simple things you can do to stay in the flow while you are breastfeeding. For Part Four, radiant circuits are introduced as wonderful ways for you to enhance the bond and attachment that you are growing with your baby.

In Part Five there are two different approaches, the Five Rhythms and Four Sensory Types, for enriching your relationship by understanding how different energy styles leave their mark on how we relate to each other. Part Six offers a delicious protocol called the Brazilian Toe Technique, which you do together with your partner, that calms the nervous system and could equally have been in Part Five on relationships, but that was already jam-packed with energy-medicine healing. Energy medicine is the way of the future, and with your well-being in mind, I am thrilled to be able to offer many healing tools for managing the fourth trimester.

As this book is coming from a strengths-based perspective, we need to celebrate the strengths that women bring to parenthood. Mothers want to be seen as women while acknowledging their interconnectedness with their babies, a both/and experience, not an either/or. The fourth trimester is a challenging time that needs to be supported by family, friends, health care providers, and the community. However, most women have only a limited awareness about the fourth trimester. I hope to fill in the blanks with the content of this book, a holistic guide for parents to thrive in the fourth trimester.

As you work your way through the book, I want to encourage you to believe in yourself and claim your power as a parent. I hope you can find your sense of humor in the process! Most of all, it is my fervent desire to help you **simplify the everyday experience** of new parenthood so that you can enjoy it more. Blessed be.

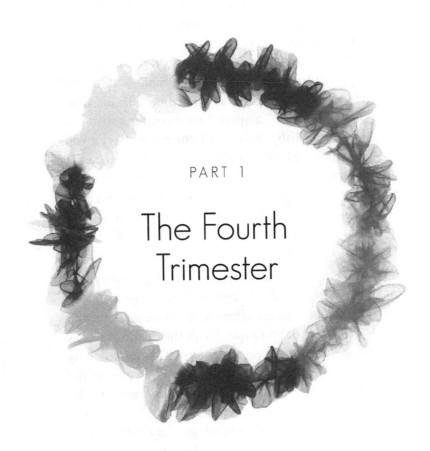

PART 1

The Fourth Trimester

PART 1 INTRODUCTION

Congratulations! The birth is finished, your baby is born, and you are now parents. You've stepped over the threshold that transforms your life forever. If you are still pregnant, this is your future. The next few months will present a whole range of new experiences with steep learning curves for you to master. With a little bit of grace and a lot of support, you might just find that the transition to parenthood is fulfilling as well as challenging. Some people call this time the "babymoon," a special moment for getting to know your baby. It's like a honeymoon, when you are alone with your partner, getting to know each other in that special cocoon of love. It is a pause in life when you can allow yourself to relax with your baby while floating on the love hormone (oxytocin) that establishes and strengthens the connection between you and your baby.

If you choose to give yourself the luxury of focused bonding time, and not race to get "back to normal," you (and your partner, if you have one) will truly benefit, and so will your baby. Keeping with the theme of simplifying life, here is important information for reducing your levels of stress. This Part is an overview of the first three months after birth for everyone in the family, and topics are presented very briefly because they will be covered in much greater depth later on, such as hormones (Part 2), breastfeeding (Part 3), bonding and attachment (Part 4), and relationships (Part 5).

I first used the term "the fourth trimester" in the 1980s in my classes and workshops as a certified childbirth educator. There is so much dynamic change going on during the three-month period from birth to 12 weeks, focused on integrating the baby, and all the new changes and roles that occur once a baby is born into the family. Substantial adjustments and the arduous amount of time invested in caregiving can be shocking to new parents, which is why we need social support to recover from birth while adapting to a new normal. When compared to the level of care and concern that pregnant women receive in the prenatal period, the postpartum period is often an overlooked time that parents muddle through. This is beginning to change with the American College of Obstetricians and Gynecologists (ACOG) 2018 Opinion statement redefining postpartum care as an ongoing process of the fourth trimester, rather than a single visit to the obstetric provider at 4 to 6 weeks postpartum. I discussed the ACOG statement in the Introduction.

These proposed changes in the provision of care reflect the lack of timely and maternal-focused health care in the postpartum period. Many women feel unprepared for the kinds of common health issues that happen, or whom to contact, resulting in unmet needs. When health issues pop up as mothers are adjusting to the demands of motherhood, this can have lasting consequences. We need to see the mother and baby as a dyad (something that consists of two elements/parts), a psychobiological connection requiring coordinated care that views the mother/baby as a mutually dependent unit that is behaviorally and physiologically intertwined. Matters like breast-feeding are poorly addressed in a system where the division of care comes from different health care providers – obstetric caregivers for mothers and pediatricians for infants. We need collaborative care between medical and other postpartum services that help mothers manage the normal postpartum challenges.

Women often encounter barriers in coping with their new reality and say the medical guidance that they do receive needs to be more nuanced and achievable. Perinatal mental health is one area where there needs to be more personalized care—not one size fits all. When screening identifies a need, there needs to be a pathway for treatment, and all too often there is none in place. Communication about women's physiological health, emotional well-being, and personal preferences are crucial to capturing women who are struggling. We need to affirm women as the experts about their babies, even when they are not experts on their postpartum health. Framing the transition to parenthood in terms of the whole family's broader situation is a more holistic approach to postpartum care. This book looks holistically at the non-medical aspects of the challenges embedded in the fourth trimester.

CHAPTER 1

Your Physical Recovery and Health

What is the Fourth Trimester?

The childbearing year consists of the nine months of pregnancy, and the first three months after birth, and the fourth trimester is the culmination of the childbearing year that starts with birth and finishes when the baby is 3 months old. It's called the fourth trimester because the kinds of adjustments that are taking place are as intense and significant as the trimesters of pregnancy, in all respects. Similar to pregnancy, the greatest changes and impact will be on the mother, but the partner, relationship, and baby are experiencing significant adjustments as well. The fourth trimester is the time it takes to fully integrate this new being into the fold. It is happening during a period of great challenge, as each member of the group is feeling needy, insecure, uncertain, and vulnerable. As a family, the different sets of needs are often at odds with each other. It is a great leap of faith to know that your family can emerge stronger and more whole through this journey together. In the midst of all the confusion and chaos of newborn parenting, a sense of cohesiveness is developing that will allow the whole family to feel connected and loved. We come out of the womb of our experience and into the light at the end of the tunnel, and the tunnel seems to go on forever—something resembling birth itself.

After birth, even though the umbilical cord has been severed, there are many times when it feels like the connection is still intact. The distinction between mother and baby is still vague; where does the mother end and baby begin? As a new mother, your self-representation changes from birth onwards. You are learning who you are in your new role, or the expansion of your role if you have other children. By the end of the fourth trimester, you can differentiate yourself from your child and feel more independent and integrated into the role of mother. This is true, whether this baby is your first or your fifth.

Mother's Experience, Recovery, and Physical Comfort Measures

The postpartum period is an overlooked area of need. As you wrestle with the task of integrating this experience, this person, and motherhood into the complexity of your life, you are encountering enormous physical changes in your body, surpassed only by the birth process itself in swiftness and speed. During pregnancy, the changes were incremental, but now the body changes are dramatic.

Lochia Discharge and Flow

For several weeks, you will have a lochia discharge. Lochia is the bleeding of the thickened endometrium (the lining of the uterus) as it heals, particularly, the site where the placenta was attached to the uterus. The blood flow will start out strong, dark red, and heavy, and then will taper off within a week to ten days. The lochia discharge will turn brown, and then get lighter as time goes by until it is just a dark stain, which will also lighten. You can judge your activity level on the flow of blood. If you are doing too much, you will continue to bleed red. If the bleeding has subsided, any fresh red blood reappearing is telling you that you are pushing your limits and need to slow down. This is avoidable when you pace yourself. The blood flow is a better barometer of how you are doing than the way you feel, which can be deceptively well.

For the first week, when the flow is heavy, using hospital-size sanitary pads is a good idea (they are much larger and effective in absorbing the flow). Some mothers prefer switching to tampons after the first week. However, the NHS in the UK and ACOG in the U.S. recommend waiting until your six-week check. One consideration in using tampons concerns whether you have lost a lot of muscular tone in the pelvic floor, making it uncomfortable to hold a tampon in place due to the loss of muscular control. This was something I encountered after my daughter's birth, and my pelvic floor had collapsed. Trying to wear tampons only caused irritation at the entrance to the vagina when the tampon slipped out of position because my muscles were so weak. The good news is that I did regain that control after many weeks of doing my Kegels (see below). There could be less chance of infection due to external bacteria. However, there is also the opposite argument; tampons work like a wick and pull germs up into the uterus. Since bleeding will continue for some weeks, tampon use could be the way to go. Another advantage is that you can go without panties to accelerate the healing process for your perineum. For people who prefer wearing external pads for vaginal bleeding, it would then be possible to switch to the size and capacity that is normal for you after a week.

Perineal Hygiene

When I had my first baby in the hospital, I was given a perineal bottle that was used to rinse the perineum (the skin between the vagina and anus) when I went to the toilet. It was a squeegee bottle that was aimed at the perineum and poured water on the area before the flow of urine. This was helpful to wash off the blood and urine before it felt comfortable enough to wipe the area with toilet paper. The warm water felt very relaxing on the stitches and the entire area, and when I was having my next baby in a birth center, I sent my husband on a mission to get me a peri-bottle from the local hospital. If that is still available in the hospital, take advantage of it. If it is not, I suggest that you get a squirt bottle for the same purpose in a pharmacy or other retailer who sells them. Alternatively, you can put a jug of warm water by the toilet, which will serve the same purpose of cleaning and relaxing the perineum.

Stitches

The stitches will be uncomfortable for a while, and the harder the surface you sit on, the better, because there will be less strain on the sit bones (ischial tuberosities) or pulling of the stitches. Even if you haven't had stitches, the perineum will be tender for a while as things heal in the vaginal area. Perineal tissues are bruised by birth, even over an intact

Kegel Exercises: Pelvic Floor Control

I cannot remember during which pregnancy I learned about doing Kegels to tone the pelvic floor, but I believe it was during my Lamaze classes with Elizabeth Bing, one of the founders of the ASPO/Lamaze organization (American Society for Psychoprophylaxis in Obstetrics), now Lamaze International'. Exercising the pelvic floor became known in the U.S. as Kegel exercises based on the work of Arnold Kegel, an American gynecologist who studied the structure and function of the muscles of the perineum. Kegels are a non-surgical treatment for relaxation of the pelvic floor, in which a person can contract the muscles by lifting and then releasing the muscles in much the same way as starting and stopping the flow of urine (which would be relaxing and then contracting the pelvic floor). He developed a device called a perineometer, which his patients used to strengthen the tone of the pelvic floor, and he had a 93% cure rate.

You can find lots of references for Kegels in a Google search. Recently, I was giving a presentation about the postpartum period to a British group of mothers and midwives, and they had no idea of what Kegels were, so I think it's limited to American birth culture. However, I did see a website in the UK offering 21st-century devices for exercising the pelvic floor called Kegel8. As I said above, when my pelvic floor collapsed after my daughter's birth (in which my 10.5 lb. baby was in the vaginal canal for a couple of hours), it was doing Kegels for weeks on end that repaired the situation. When I went to see the midwife at six weeks, and she told me to do a Kegel, my efforts were futile. Nothing happened! That told me I had to get to work.

During pregnancy, the figure 8 muscles that comprise the pelvic floor become relaxed, including the sphincter muscles surrounding the urethra, vagina, and anus. When you pull up the muscles, you are contracting all the sphincters at the same time. As a birth educator, I would present a variety of ways of doing Kegels that increased the level of control that mothers had over the pelvic floor. In addition to lifting and releasing, they could lift, hold for a second, and then release. Or they could hold it for three counts or lift to the count of three and release to the count of three. By developing tone during pregnancy, when the hammock-like pelvic floor is under pressure from the weight of the pregnancy, causing it to sag a little, this helps the pelvic floor return to normal more quickly after birth. One pleasurable way to improve the muscle tone of the pelvic floor is to contract the muscles during intercourse when you can get feedback from your partner, who will feel it (once you are ready to resume penetrative sex). When the pelvic floor remains loose, this can lead to stress incontinence, prolapse, and sexual dysfunction, so decide now to make the effort to strengthen the pelvic floor. If you did 10 Kegels at every meal, you would be well on your way to getting your tone back. I did.

Hormonal Shifts

The birth of the placenta precipitates tremendous hormonal shifts, as estrogen and progesterone levels plummet (these were being produced by the placenta). It shouldn't escalate past blues when the mother is being adequately nurtured and supported. Another feature of the blues is the anticlimax after the birth high. After so much waiting to meet your baby, it is surprising how many women feel the sadness of it being over far too fast. The hormones are working to help every cell and organ in the body to return to their pre-pregnancy state, and their involvement with emotions may leave you feeling vulnerable. Your feelings, both positive and negative, may be very close to the surface at this time.

Rest and Exercise

Even though you may be feeling great because you experienced natural childbirth, you still need plenty of rest. You need total rest for the first two or three days, to give your body a chance to recover, and more if you've had a cesarean section. After that, you need regular rest periods every single day. This doesn't often happen after the first birth, but experienced mothers know the importance of this rest. The amount of rest you have in the beginning is directly related to your ability to avoid depression later. Sleep deprivation is a known risk factor for perinatal mental illness. Recent research has revealed that depression is the outcome of ongoing stress and the inflammation caused by stress hormones circulating throughout the body. Women are vulnerable to postpartum depression during this period of restoring the body to its non-pregnant state due to the added reproductive hormones shifting. If a mother has not had enough rest, this condition is exacerbated and can become a serious medical issue when it becomes severe and persistent. Observing a rest period after birth is a terrific preventive measure.

While getting adequate rest is important, once you feel ready, you can offset that with some exercise. I taught postpartum exercise classes for 20 years, so I have a natural bias to encourage women to take part in classes like I offered. Exercise will speed the healing process and improve your mood. You can do some easy movements in the early days, and then find a class as the fourth trimester draws to an end. Today, there are so many options, with postpartum yoga, Pilates, stroller workouts (my daughter did this one), walking, swimming, light weight training, and cycling. If you've had a cesarean, it is wise to wait for the all-clear at six weeks.

Nutrition

You also need proper nutrition to regain your strength. That means a balanced diet of macronutrients that include protein, carbohydrates, fat, and water. Those categories should include all the food groups. Protein sources are meat, fish, poultry, eggs, dairy products, and nuts/seeds. Whole grains are cereals, bread, baked goods, and pasta. Fruits and vegetables are healthier forms of carbohydrates that are loaded with vitamins and minerals (micronutrients). Our recently developed understanding of the importance of essential fatty acids, especially the omega-3s, EPA and DHA, means that we need to consume some healthy fats to be healthy. The elements of good nutrition had changed dramatically since the days when I was teaching my pregnant clients about nutrition. But who has time to sort out this healthy eating when a baby has just been born?

The irony of the nurturing mother not nourishing herself is too common of an occurrence. It is almost as if feeding the baby is going to feed the mother by some kind of osmosis. Or in real terms, the mother does not create time to feed herself after all the feeding rituals for the baby are done. This is, paradoxically, another way to feed depression. Better you should feed yourself than suffer the consequences of malnutrition or just the everyday periods of low blood sugar.

In the beginning, there is the excitement of wanting to share the arrival of the new baby with friends and relatives. Those visits are surprisingly tiring, and it is a good idea to ration the time spent with people visiting.

Having visitors can be beneficial if you request that everyone who visits brings food ready to eat. You might get tired, but at least you'll be well-fed. Being well-rested and well-fed restores a sense of normalcy in the midst of so much change. But remember, life is different now. You cannot expect things to go "back to normal" when normal is now different. Eat a well-balanced diet over the course of the day because you would be hard pressed to do it in any one meal. Being a mother is not being a martyr. Your needs, the baby's needs, and your partner's needs are the priority, in that order, more or less.

Hydration

Remember to stay hydrated during this time. It's essential for your basic health and the production of breast milk. Having lots of fluids throughout the day will help you to stay strong with all the demands being made on your energy and will also help with mental clarity. Every time you sit down to feed your baby, there should be a glass of something for you to drink too. Ideally, it would be water, and this is a great time to increase your intake of water. As with food, getting enough to drink is a challenge to new mothers, so enlisting the help of others can make a real difference. Let others know you need to be drinking to keep your levels of hydration healthy because the last thing you need during this time is to become dehydrated. Some of the symptoms of dehydration are headaches, sleepiness, difficulty concentrating, low energy, and digestive issues. Since the body is at least 60% water (and some would say more), replenishing your fluids is a daily matter. Put reminders around the house so you don't forget. And while you're at it, put reminders up to eat too. You will feel better for the effort to eat and drink, and if you can arrange for help with this from your partner, relatives, other children, and friends, even better.

Breast Engorgement and Soreness

In those first few days after birth, your milk becomes more abundant. Depending on how freely you nurse, it could be the second, third, or fourth day. If you nurse frequently, your engorgement will be minimal, if non-existent. However, if you nurse on a schedule, you're likely to feel much more discomfort as the breasts fill with fluids. If you experience sore nipples, which could continue for a couple of weeks, it could impede the breastfeeding connection. Even if increase of light sleep, and the suppression of rapid-eye-movement (REM) sleep and less REM sleep affects our mood and energy levels. I believe this is nature's way of preparing women to wake up when their babies cry in the night. Having rest periods while pregnant can reduce the impact of sleep loss after the baby is born, although so many women work right up until their due date that this can be difficult to arrange.

Nursing and keeping your baby close by during the night lightens the load since you can doze during feeding and you don't have to rouse yourself fully. There's the advantage of nursing the baby in a different position (lying down), emptying all the milk ducts on the sides as well. However, there are exceptions to this strategy for women who have a hard time sleeping near the baby making typical baby noises as it sleeps. Sidecar co-sleepers are a great invention, and I would have loved to have had one during my childbearing years. However, they may not work for the woman who is sensitive to noise. Her light sleep patterns may be easily disrupted, making matters worse.

Power Sleep

It has become something of a cliché to tell mothers to sleep when their babies sleep, but it is wisdom that has stood the test of time. Having even short naps can reduce your sleep debt.

Strategies that can help with fatigue:

▶ avoiding caffeinated drinks in the evening,

▶ going to sleep earlier, if possible, and developing a bedtime ritual that helps you relax, and

▶ adjusting your social life by turning down invitations or going home early.

Understand that when you experience a deep sleep state, your body is producing healthy levels of prolactin that will make breastfeeding easier. Be smart about your sleep debt and notice when you are drowsy and alert. Unattended sleep debt can have a detrimental impact on carbohydrate metabolism, endocrine function, and other adverse effects on your health. Keeping your sleep debt low, by getting extra sleep to make up for short nights, will help you decrease sleep deprivation.

Until sleeping through the night happens, you can get cranky with lack of sleep, which further complicates your emotional condition. I admire attachment parents who practice nighttime parenting without losing their sense of humor. Even the most sophisticated mother has her moments of insecurity and uncertainty after a new baby is born. For someone doing this for the first time, with no previous experience, those insecurities can dominate your perceptions of how you're doing. Having a doula to mother you is vital for building confidence; hiring a postpartum doula is one of the best ideas for navigating the early days after birth. Dana Raphael, in her book *The Tender Gift: Breastfeeding* (1976), introduced me to the concept of a "doula" over 40 years ago and also to the process of *matrescence*, which is not well-understood in our culture and hardly supported.

Matrescence

Matrescence is the process of becoming a mother in the full sense of the experience on all levels of experience. It means fully taking on the role and seeing how it fits, recognizing the areas that require adjustments and making them. In a society without a built-in support system, it can mean going it alone, which can be daunting when mothers are discharged from the hospital within hours of giving birth. The normalization of what was once "early discharge" means the mother is expected to take full responsibility for mothering with little training and less support, and before her readiness to assume the task. This expectation for new mothers involves sending our mothers home seriously lacking in confidence and skill.

Raphael said, "The common denominator for success in breastfeeding is the assurance of some degree of help from some specific person for a definite period after childbirth" (Raphael, 1976, p. 141). The presence of a caring individual, whose sole purpose is to mother the mother by confirmation, reassurance, and support, allows the mother to establish the rhythm of sucking and letting down that is crucial in the first weeks after birth. The *doula* (the Greek word for servant) is an experienced mother who comes into the home and assists by cooking, helping with other children, holding the baby so that the mother can have a shower or do other non-baby related tasks, offering breastfeeding support and counseling, and tending to other chores or errands that need attention.

The goddesses whose glory was defined by their relationships to others (wife, mother, daughter) were considered vulnerable goddesses. Those who were independent were the virgin goddesses, meaning they were whole unto themselves, not the mundane use of the word today.

The vulnerability of new motherhood is a lesson to embrace during the fourth trimester. Those accustomed to clear focus in their work or career experiences can have a difficult time making this adjustment to free-flowing openness. Life loses its crisp focus, which feels like a loss of control, and that can be threatening to women who have been groomed to take a sharp view of life. In the bigger picture, this is a brief period in life, despite the impression that time seems to have slowed down to the minute (which began during labor itself). This prepares you for living in "baby time," when you are on the baby's schedule, and the best thing you can do is take life one moment at the time. When we let go and surrender into the moment, we can accept ourselves in our new role. Our self-esteem rises, our confidence expands, and our trust deepens.

Time to Adjust

Bringing a new baby home is exciting and overwhelming at times, especially if this is a first. There are emotional adjustments to the whole new experience, with awesome responsibility, protective love, and fears for its health and safety. There are huge relationship adjustments to this new situation in which you will be interacting in very different ways as you absorb a child into the family. If there are other children, you may feel the pull between your need to take care of the baby when your older child needs attention too. You are learning to do so many new things—like breastfeeding, diapering, bathing, and settling a baby to sleep—and all of this is on-the-job training. I like to think of this book as the manual that doesn't come when a baby is born.

You are also forging a connection with a new person, and there is a paradox to the bonding and separation that are features of the fourth trimester. The postpartum period is the first step in a long and gradual process of separation that is unfolding over time, dramatically initiated by birth. That separation from one into two necessitates a reunion between mother and infant for the baby to thrive. Bonding, contrary to what one hears, is not always an instant love affair. It can take days and weeks to form that connection between you and the baby. Bonding, which we will discuss in Part 4, is an ongoing process that is best served by a restful postpartum period.

The 40 Days

Around the world, there are traditions for postpartum women, cultural norms that facilitate recovery. They are most frequently referred to as "the 40 days," which happens to be roughly six weeks. During this time, the mother is safely sequestered in either her own home or in a special location designed for postpartum women. She is attended by her female kin, who provide support and assistance with the baby and take responsibility for the upkeep of the space. The purpose is to give the new mother time to slowly recover from birth and enjoy a cozy time building a loving relationship with her newborn, as the babymoon mentioned previously. The 40 days also takes into account the sensitivity of the newborn, and during this time, the baby is protected in a sacred environment with the mother and intimate family, when this takes place at home. Partners and siblings are cultivating their relationship with the newborn during this sensitive time when reverence for the 40 days after birth is upheld. Family and friends assist with the household, the rest of the family, and childcare. This is also done by postpartum doulas these days, who can help to create a sacred atmosphere during the postpartum period.

International Traditions

In Asian cultures, such as China and Vietnam, the time is often called "doing the month," or "sitting the month," and there are special centers that provide new mothers with some pampered seclusion during this time of postpartum confinement. It's generally for 30 days and has prescribed foods and restrictions on activities designed to help promote contraction of the uterus, promote lactation, and heal the perineum.

The Japanese have a similar custom of *ansei*, or peace and quiet, to help with the recuperation process for a period after giving birth. These postpartum houses can be expensive, costing thousands of dollars, which is probably why the time is shortened to 30 days. A "proper" confinement can be between 45 and 60 days long. The emphasis is on warmth, and as we will see in the Part on hormones, there is probably a connection between this warmth and the flow of oxytocin. Foods are consumed to facilitate the recovery process and include special additives, like eucommia bark and goji berries, known to purge the uterus, and adzuki beans are believed to reduce swelling. Cold foods are forbidden during the month because they are believed to slow down the involution process. Foods believed to cool down the body's energy flow include cabbage and watermelon.

Greek customs adhere to the 40 days, "fortying," and this confinement happens at home, after which the baby is symbolically taken to church for the first time at the end of the mother's postpartum period, and the mother asks for a special blessing. The modern interpretations of this traditional practice include an unimpeded establishment of breastfeeding, bonding time between parent and child, and protecting the undeveloped immune system of the newborn.

In India, the tradition of confinement and recuperation is called *Jaappa* in Hindi, and a special diet is involved that facilitates milk production and increases hemoglobin levels. There are issues of pollution, or impurity, in this culture due to the childbirth process, and sex is not allowed. The mother is exempted from household chores and other matters of everyday life. The father would be purified with a ritual bath before visiting the mother in confinement.

Mothering the Mother

These examples of cultures that provide this period of seclusion for new mothers is a far cry from the absence of postpartum support in most English-speaking countries. These traditions are also common in South America, where it is called *la cuarentena* (quarantine), and the Middle East. Maybe the word confinement makes it seem unappealing, but there is wisdom in this approach to the postpartum period. It is nurturing and nourishing to be looked after at a time when your vulnerability is at its peak. Anything that will facilitate the symbiotic relationship between you and your baby is a way to avoid suffering for both of you. It is a way of mothering the mother, which we will explore more in later chapters, and it offers the space for you to do nothing else but bond with your baby. Forty days may not be realistic if you have other children, or have to work to pay bills, but it's a matter of attitude to what's expected of women, or what women expect of themselves, in the postpartum period. Unrealistic expectations of what's possible can do a woman in.

If the 40 days tradition were embraced in our society, there could be much more ease and flow during this transition, rather than anxiety and depression for not having met the harsh expectations of what "should" be. One thing that I have suggested to new parents over the years is to create a "Contract for Hours" for friends and family to complete. One book that will help you do this is Michelle Peterson's, *7 Sisters for Seven Days*. This acknowledges the support that people want to give, and also clearly specifies which type of help would be most useful in advance: help taking older children to after-school activities, bringing cooked meals, talking on the phone, and any variety of tasks that others are happy to do for you.

Asking for help is a challenge for many people, but when others ask, "how can I help?" you have a list of suggestions that people can sign up for. And they will. A recent blog post by Svea Boyda-Vikander had some great ideas for alternatives to baby shower gifts: gift certificates to restaurants that deliver, housework coupons, and a stay at a posh hotel (on the more extravagant end) rather than registries in stores. "I would like to see partners and families allocate some funds to this period; for it to be acknowledged as the special, difficult, tear-filled, milky mess of a time that it is," she said (http://birthwithoutfearblog.com/2012/10/21/mothering-the-mother-40-days-of-rest/).

On a more esoteric level, some believe that when the child is in the womb, you share physical functions and subtle energies, as you are blended in one aura. The separation of the auras happens when the umbilical cord is cut, and for those who are sensitive to energy, this can be a shock. Over the next three years, the auras will become autonomous, but during this time of subtle connection, the baby is focused primarily on the mother, while the father/partner provides essential security and support for both.

it is contact with another body that is the physicality that feels safe. Our culture is only beginning to recognize this requirement as being fundamental to healthy development. Attachment parenting is the movement that has grown from an acceptance of this actuality. Babywearing has grown in popularity with a whole host of slings, carriers, and wraps to keep the baby close.

Errors of Our Past and Present: The Importance of Contact

Close contact is essential for stimulation and nourishment. The baby becomes the center of attention during the fourth trimester, disproportionately so, to the detriment of the mother. We make judgments on how much touch and contact is acceptable, a trend that was started in the early 20th century and revived at the beginning of the 21st century. The first wave of restriction around contact with the baby originated with John B. Watson, who wrote *Psychological Care of Infant and Child* in 1928, the original parenting guide that warned against giving the baby too much love and affection. He promoted a business-like attitude between mother and baby, based on his radical behaviorist approach to psychology, advocating for an efficient child rearing process that warned against holding the baby in the parent's lap. He coined the phrase "spoiling your baby."

Over the years, Watson's book and theories came under critical scrutiny and were discredited for the degree of emotional detachment it endorsed. Some would say his theories were based on his difficult circumstances in growing up without a father, who abandoned the family when Watson was 13. His views were reflective of the times, but his granddaughter, actress Mariette Hartley, wrote her own scathing personal review of what life was like growing up in his family in her book, *Breaking the Silence,* in 1990 (a new edition came out in 2010).

The 20th-century tendency toward "expert advice" has culminated in a recent book that has become a bible for some new mothers in the 21st century, *The (New) Contented Little Baby Book,* by Gina Ford. This is a book to either love or hate and has generated quite a lively debate as to its usefulness in imposing a routine on life with a baby. The author is *not* a mother and based her book on her experience as a maternity nurse working in a hospital, which explains the extreme regimentation she promotes. Someone who hasn't had the postpartum experience of mothering has no credibility with me, and I'm alarmed that more mothers don't protest this when struggling to apply the approach her book encourages. The routine is more important than the baby, and the daily schedule is almost militaristic in its precision. This is not how energy flows in the fourth trimester and trying to conform to such a program is unnecessary pressure on new parents. I have a problem with any methodology that advocates letting a child cry for long periods of time to learn how to sleep through the night (I will return to the subject of sleep training in Part 4). This will break the spirit of any new baby who is struggling to make so many profound adjustments to life on earth. The drama of the transition is challenging enough without adding this insensitive "training" at such a tender stage of life.

All the baby requires is the sensuous contact with the mother's body, to which it has already structured points of similarity that allow it to interact with its new earthly matrix. Joseph Chilton Pearce talks about this in his classic book, *The Magical Child*. He describes how the baby accomplishes an important step in the cycle of competence, namely practice with the possibility. If the mother is not available, this work does not get done, and intelligence and development slow down. Gina Ford and Joseph Chilton Pearce are miles apart in what they have to offer new parents.

How Babies Interact

As time goes by, and you and baby become more in tune with each other, the innate sociality of the baby is activated. Smiling begins by 6 weeks (give or take a week or two), and often much sooner. It is not gas (wind), as previous generations believed. My last child smiled the day after he was born for a friend who came to visit, and we discovered his dimple that was named after her. Premature babies take longer to smile, and it is useful to count six weeks from the original due date. In the book *Your Amazing Newborn* (1998) by Phyllis and Marshall Klaus, the extraordinary acuity of most of the newborn's senses is described. We know that babies are born with well-developed senses and the intrinsic ability to utilize them.

The reference about babies sleeping 90% of the time is based on research done in the mid-20th century on the six states of consciousness in babies around sleep and wakefulness. The two sleep states are quiet sleep and active sleep. The three wakeful states are quiet-alert, active-alert, and crying. The last state is drowsiness, the state between wakefulness and sleep. My concern is for those new parents whose baby does not sleep 90% of the time, as they are bound to think something is wrong with their babies, or wrong with them, while they are in a heightened place of vulnerability. To put it into perspective, it is important to know that this is just for the first two weeks.

Babies do smile, and they do it as their first social expression. It's quite effective in keeping parents engaged. After that wears thin, around 3 months, babies start to laugh and giggle. This is even more engaging and assures the contact that the baby needs, both physically and socially. Babies are affected by the mother's increasing levels of tension as the day goes on. They feel it energetically and become reactive to it. The witching hours start around 4:00 to 5:00 pm and continue through to about 8:00 pm or so. You are tense and tired, and the baby responds by crying. Unfortunately, your partner usually comes home just around this time when things are disintegrating and is asked to take over. This brings us to the father's or partner's experience of the fourth trimester.

Father's or Partner's Experience

This is the father's first opportunity to fully hold and caress his child, and to meet it face to face and have his first personal and sensuous contact with his baby. There is a qualitative difference to feeling the baby move through several layers of mother's abdominal tissues and feeling this baby in his arms. The father can now literally carry some of the load—he can hold, play with, change, and soothe the baby. This may not be opportune at the witching hour, when the father is bombarded with the full responsibility on arrival at home. And speaking of responsibility, the dad is feeling more burdened by his increased responsibility as the breadwinner in the family, with his partner now on maternity leave. The father is often the only one who is working and bringing home income, even if it is temporary, yet he wants to have his intimate time with the baby too, to experience bonding with his child as a satisfying involvement. He may be feeling torn in learning how to divide his time between work and family, and where his priorities are being set. In some cases, it *isn't* the father who is the breadwinner in the family, and this can initiate a very different dynamic in the household.

It is a good idea to keep in mind that partners need some babying too. Because sexual relations might be on the backburner during the early stage of the postpartum period, when everything seems to be focused on the baby, partners need to feel loved and cared for too. Cuddling can be a substitute for lovemaking until the time and energy for sexual relations returns. In Part 2, we will examine how the father is also experiencing hormonal adjustments in parallel with his pregnant and postpartum partner.

Changing Gender Roles

Dad's culture has stereotypical roles for the father to accept or reject in defining himself as a father (there are no stereotypes of second mothers/ female partners or gay parents yet). These stereotypes bring up all his insecurities about who he wants to be as a father, and this may also reflect the kind of fathering he had. Since he is feeling moderately sleep deprived as well, these insecurities become magnified, and he feels out of sorts. He doesn't feel quite right in the home environment leading to dichotomies: my world, which is the workplace, and her world at home with the baby. Some women have told me that this assumption has sexist overtones to it and is not always accurate. Being more comfortable or confident at work, and less insecure, many fathers overcompensate by spending more time at work. What does this do to the relationship? It puts a strain on the dynamics of intimacy, which is one of the reasons The Birth Empowerment Workshop' places so much emphasis on communication and relationship before birth. This helps couples move through this highly charged trimester without creating distance between them. They become a duet.

Relationships

There is a true shift in emphasis during the fourth trimester regarding the relationship. The pressure of having almost no time alone to recharge the love for each other is significant. All the energy directed towards the baby leaves the relationship suffering depletion of reserves. Sometimes jealousy rises to the surface for both the mother and father. She is jealous that he gets to leave every day and accomplish something in the world. He is jealous of her ability to nurture her baby at the breast, a form of nurturing that excludes him. He is also jealous of the amount of time and attention the baby is receiving; he used to have mother's undivided attention when it was just "the two of us." Fathers with older children see added distance between him and his mate, with each focusing on different children.

Any siblings will be connecting to the new baby as well, each bringing their personalities into the fray, especially when stepchildren are involved. When a couple has taken the time to nurture their relationship before birth, then these difficulties need only be transient. A wonderful book on how to stay connected in the transition to parenthood is *Becoming Us: 8 Steps to Grow a Family that Thrives* by Elly Taylor (2014). It is full of excellent strategies for working as a team, and for understanding the perspective of the partner during this challenging time for the relationship. I will review this book in greater detail in Part 5 on relationships. I've been so personally excited by this work that I became a Certified Becoming Us™ Facilitator.

Intimacy

The postpartum ban on lovemaking puts additional strains on intimacy, which is unfortunate, because intercourse is only one form of pleasure, and there are other ways of pleasuring each other during this time if there is energy. It is a good idea to wait until the postpartum check-up before having penetrative sex, but it's not absolute. This will give you an idea of how well things have healed down below, and how comfortable you are likely to be. When women are breastfeeding, the prolactin that is produced by the body causes the vagina to be dry, and this can be alleviated using lubricating jelly, such as K-Y jelly. The first penetration is likely to be uncomfortable, especially after stitches that make the area tighter and more inflamed than normal. Often, mothers have so little energy at the end of the day that they are unable to give to a sexual relationship, which put it on the backburner in the first place. They can be feeling "touched out" by the intimate contact with the baby all day. I particularly like this quote from Elizabeth Bing and Libby Colman's classic book, *Making Love During Pregnancy:*

> In the early weeks after resuming sex, the baby herself did not intrude on our relations, but my exhaustion and discomfort did. The tenderness from the episiotomy lasted a good deal longer than six weeks, and this surprised me. More importantly, my total absorption in the baby and mothering drastically cut my interest and desire for sex. After spending the day with a non-napping, non-stop baby... by evening I had absolutely nothing left to give. All I wanted was to be left alone, go to sleep or just regroup myself – to replenish the patient, love-giving attention I had used up during the day. At first, I thought I was alone in this to the extent I felt it...But friends have since told me that they felt the same – never watching so much mindless TV as they did from childbirth to about 3 months. And I too found that midway through the third month I had integrated the baby into my life enough to return to a normal (non-baby related) conversation and sex (Bing & Colman, 1977, pp. 148-149).

Parenting a Newborn

Newborn parenting is a trial-and-error process, and we all make mistakes along the way. That is the best way to learn, as it is human to make mistakes, and it is in the correction that the lesson is truly learned. When I was training in hypnosis, our instructor told us that all pilots, when they are learning to fly a plane, are required to stall, to learn how to correct that situation. A mother needs to find peers with experience who she can reach out to and allow that support to bolster her self-confidence as she adjusts to being a parent in the here and now. What your mother did in her generation won't necessarily apply in yours. Please let yourself receive support in as many ways as you can because it comes in all shapes and sizes: friendship, and physical, emotional, practical, and financial support.

Don't make the mistake of comparing your baby to others. Each baby will learn on its trajectory, some physically, others linguistically, and still others, socially. It all balances out around the age of 3 anyway, but you could make yourself miserable if your baby is not doing what others do at the usual time. Einstein did not speak until he was 4 years old.

Here's a link to a quick video, created by Adriana Lozada, that can add a little lightness to the newborn parenting experience by giving some perspective on how a day in the life of a newborn works. She calls it *Life with a Newborn: Why It's So Hard to Take a Shower*: https://www.youtube.com/watch?v=oQt90SHj6iY&feature=youtu.be.

CHAPTER 4

Postpartum W.E.L.L.N.E.S.S. Plan

At the start of this book, I talked about the importance of simplifying your life during the postpartum period. One way of doing that is by creating a Postpartum Wellness Plan as a means of navigating the normal challenges that are a natural feature of those early days and weeks after birth. A postpartum plan is just as important as a birth plan; after all, it lasts a lot longer than the baby's birth. The acronym that I created around "WELLNESS" covers the basics that will help you make all the necessary adjustments for recovery and parenting that dominate the experience. WELLNESS stands for the following:

(W) = We

(E) = Energy medicine

(L) = Lovingkindness

(L) = Less is more

(N) = New normal

(E) = Expectations

(S) = Self-care

(S) = Support

We

Protecting your partnership as you become parents is crucial for making life much simpler, as the birth of a baby brings so much change with it that we often take the stress out on our partners. The last thing you need is to alienate your partner when the going gets rough because it feels bad to not have the loving support you need in those moments. You want to be on the same page when it comes to managing the everyday reality of the transition to parenthood. Part 5 on relationships will explain the importance of prioritizing your relationship so that there are empathy and compassion keeping you connected with each other. "We" is also about the family that you are creating. Your "we" has expanded to include another little person in your life. Welcome your parent self, as Elly Taylor says in her *8 Steps of the Parenthood Adventure*. Both of you are going through your transitions, as well as a major relationship transition in which each of you will have your vulnerabilities. Turning towards each other for love and support makes a huge difference in those early days as you are trying on the role of parent. Respect that each of you will do things slightly differently, and that's fine. Avoid right and wrong interpretations, because that increases stress and makes the other person feel less capable. Be there for each other and work together. I love the metaphor of being a duet, where each of you can sing your part, but there is harmony in the sound both of you create together. Nurture your partnership.

Energy Medicine

The four principles of energy medicine are the foundation of healing with energy: 1) energy wants to move, 2) energy needs space to move, 3) the health of the body reflects the health of its energies, and 4) the body's energies are interconnected. One of the best things about working with energy medicine (which will be introduced further in the next chapter) is that it offers so many opportunities for healing yourself and doesn't require anyone else to do it for you. You are your healer. You can also visit an energy medicine practitioner for even more yummy treatments, but that's an indulgence that might not be possible in the weeks after birth.

The common actuality of low energy in those early weeks when sleep deprivation is the norm can be rectified by doing the Daily Energy Routine

(DER) that will be described in the next chapter. I do this every evening, and I find that when I don't do it, I don't sleep as well. Other people do it in the morning to get themselves off to a good start in the day. Keeping your energy flowing through the various techniques that are described at the end of each Part puts you in control. What's wonderful is the simplicity of these practices, and how effective they can be. I truly believe this is a happy medium for tuning in to your energetic needs, and I wish I had energy healing when I was having babies. The health of our energy lies in its flow, balance, and harmony, impacting on the health of the body. When the body is unhealthy, the energies are also disturbed and need to be repaired.

You can also do some of the techniques as a couple together – certainly, the DER, but also the stress-related techniques, the relationship techniques, and the one that I saved for the last chapter is a real winner. The Brazilian Toe Technique is just delightful.

Lovingkindness

When it comes to sharing love, empathy, and caring, lovingkindess is the way. It comes from the Buddhist spiritual tradition and lights the way for the journey to the heart. In the midst of the confusion that is normal in the postpartum period, we need to open our hearts to each other and to the new baby that has just arrived earth-side. Most importantly, we need to open our hearts to ourselves, with self-love and acceptance. Lovingkindness is the English translation for *Metta* practice, a meditation in which we offer care and friendship to ourselves and then to others, wishing for mental happiness, physical happiness, freedom from danger and ease of well-being. The *Metta* phrases are: "May I be free from danger," "May I have mental happiness," "May I have physical happiness," and "May I have ease of well-being" (Salzberg, 1995). This is then extended outwards to include 1) a person who is a "benefactor"; 2) a beloved friend; 3) a neutral person; and then, 4) someone with whom you have experienced conflict, sometimes called "the enemy." The happiness that we wish for ourselves becomes happiness for all. With all others, you would substitute the word "you" for I, e.g., "May you be free from danger," etc.

Understandably, you will say you have no time for meditation, and I'm not suggesting that you can. It's the essence of being kind to yourself and others that can become the atmosphere in which your family blossoms.

What you will find in the next book, *The Adverse Aftermath of Birth*, is that expectations can undermine our capacity to function or accept the new normal. I'll mention in Part 5 how we can have helpful, and unhelpful, expectations, and those unhelpful ones can really do a number on us emotionally. We have expectations about so many areas of our lives during this time frame: expectations about ourselves as parents, and about life, our relationships, ourselves, our partners, and our babies. We need to manage those expectations effectively. It would be a good exercise to write down your expectations, and if they are unhelpful, see if you can rephrase them as helpful ones. Borrowing an example from Elly Taylor's Becoming US™ training, "even though we've been having some relationship issues, this baby will bring us closer," is an unhelpful expectation. A helpful expectation might be, "even though we will feel closer in some ways, in other ways we will have new challenges to confront." It's an expectation that recognizes that your ideal of what should be needs some flexibility built into it. You can do this on your own, or you can do it as a couple. Don't let unrealistic expectations cause your descent into depression and anxiety.

Self-Care

This is a tricky one since it's common for mothers to forget to take care of themselves while they are so busy taking care of newborns. But it is essential for our physical, emotional, and mental health that we take the time to look after ourselves. That might be eating nutritious meals and snacks, and getting someone to supply or prepare those for you, staying hydrated throughout the day, especially while breastfeeding, or practicing the energy-medicine techniques, which are highly effective for managing your energy levels at this time. Finding time for a shower (remember Adriana Lozada's video) or bath might be challenging, but it's something you can do when your partner is around to hold the baby. Here's where the flexibility comes in: being able to change your normal routine to a time that works for you and the baby. So, if you are used to having your shower in the morning, maybe it will temporarily change to an evening time instead. Having "me time" is also very important when you are engaged in baby-care 24/7. And "we time" too, so you stay connected through the chaotic moments. That might just be holding hands while you watch television and rest. Even though you may not be sleeping through the night, you can catch up on your sleep debt if you take naps during the day, when the baby is resting. Don't succumb to that temptation to run around and clean up when the baby sleeps. Your rest is more important for restoring balance. Get outside and breathe in some fresh air as often as you can. It does change your frame of mind to be outside in nature, if you live where this is accessible. Even a park in the city will do. What kinds of things do you do for yourself to feel good? Maybe it's reaching out to friends by telephone. Whatever you do to promote self-care, make time for it.

Support

And finally, and last but not least, is support. It does take a village to raise a child. Parenting was not meant to be done without the love and support of our community. Once upon a time, that was the norm, in which family, community, and elders all contributed to the happy and healthy development of a new family. Within the relationship, you want to support each other as you move through the transition as "we" because part of the synergy of "we" is supporting each other. And there are so many forms of support, as mentioned previously. When I was writing my thesis for my PhD, one of the main themes was social support, along with knowledge and empowerment, and the formula was Knowledge + Support = Empowerment. This is true in birth and life after birth.

Don't be afraid to ask for help. For many people, that's a growing edge, and they find it difficult. For those who are feeling particularly vulnerable, it feels like asking for help is an admission that you are not coping. And maybe you're not. But the sooner you get help, the faster you'll feel better. If you've had a cesarean section, you have to accept assistance and support because there will be many things you're unable to do when you are post-operative. The solution? The "Contract for Hours" that I mentioned earlier. People want to support you, and if you indicate what you need in advance, people can decide how they can best respond. When I was preparing for Jasper's arrival, I had people sign up for ways they could support me with their time and efforts. One person signed up to bring us dinner. Someone else, who had also just had a baby the day after me, signed up for telephone chats. Someone signed up to take my other children to afterschool activities. Someone signed up to shop for us. Embrace support in any way it comes, for whatever your needs are. It will surely help you, and it will help those who want to be there for you, in definite and specific ways. No empty offer of help, or you struggling to decide what help you need. Make it part of your wellness plan.

How will you construct your plan around wellness? Working as a team, decide how you want to do this.

(W) Create some we time.

(E) Practice energy-medicine techniques, individually and together.

(L) Embrace the attitude of lovingkindness with each other, even when things are challenging.

(L) What can you do less of? Have less of? Decide how "less is more" works for you.

(N) Be mindful of how your normal has changed and accept this as a good thing.

(E) Share your expectations with each other and see how you can make them into helpful expectations that express your development as individuals and as a family.

(S) Do something that establishes self-care every day. You'll feel better for it, and you will bring that energy into the care you give to your baby and your partner.

(S) Get all the support that you need by speaking out. Overcome any reticence and let others help you.

Your Postpartum Wellness Plan will help you shape your lives together as parents and as a family.

CHAPTER 5

Emotions and Energy

Emotions: The Positive, the Negative, and the Roller Coaster

I could not write this book without addressing the power of emotions, as the subject is embedded in so much that is written. Some would say that our emotions are all over the place after a baby is born, as we are trying to manage all the new experiences that parenthood presents. Sometimes, it is a roller coaster: ups and downs can occur on a daily basis, especially a few days after birth when the effects of low levels of hormones impact on our mood. The transition to parenthood is a time of mixed emotions, and they can be happening at the same time. It's important to understand that the postpartum period is not all sweetness and light. Elation can be mixed with fear of the unknown. Excitement can be mixed with overwhelm. Joy is mixed with uncertainty. Our emotions are complex, and they allow us to experience the textures and colors of life as they give meaning to our lives. The key is to use our emotions wisely, so they don't destroy us (www.hearthmath.org).

Emotion is "**e**(energy in)**motion**." Emotions can drive our decisions and actions, building energy assets to add to the quality of life or energy deficits that cheat us of vitality. So often, we are at the mercy of our emotions, reacting to external events rather than making conscious choices. It's important to be able to learn how to consciously adjust our emotions to reduce our experiences of the roller coaster of emotions. We are more able than we realize to choose what we want to experience in our feeling world.

Fundamentally, emotions are neutral, and they add power to our thoughts by amplifying them. Thought, backed up by emotions, is how we create our reality in life. The world of feeling operates at a higher speed than the mind, and our emotional reactions show up in brain activity before we've had a chance to think. The more primitive parts of the brain are where the emotions are activated, and thought requires that more advanced parts of the brain are stimulated. We evaluate everything emotionally as we perceive it.

The process of experiencing emotions is biochemical and neurological, involving the heart, brain, nervous and hormonal systems (more on these in the next Part), and sensory organs. Our emotional experience is a combination of feeling sensations, associated thoughts, and biochemical reactions that shape our emotional experience. Emotions are the product of an ongoing dialogue between the body and the brain. Anger and anxiety can tighten our necks and shoulders. Fear can be felt in the stomach. Sorrow is felt in the chest. Emotions on the positive side of things—love, appreciation, compassion, and kindness—allow us to relax so our body's communication system can flow with greater harmony and efficiency.

A cascade of 1,400 different biochemicals is released by the body when it senses a stressful emotion, and negative emotions can keep the system bathed in stress hormones, which speeds up aging, and drains us of emotional resilience and physical vitality. Added on top of all that's involved in recovering from birth, the mind and body are going through a huge amount of turmoil and adjustment: all the more reason to be compassionate with ourselves at this time. Speak up when you need support. Don't assume that those around you will know what you need. If you need emotional support, ask for it from others.

Negative emotions cause the stress response to be activated, and I discuss this in detail in Part 2. The good news is that positive emotions can undo the effects of negative emotions by loosening the hold that they have on the brain and body. Positive emotions produce biochemicals that are regenerative and beneficial, and the science is there to back up ways to help regulate emotions. The HeartMath Institute (HMI) has been the leader in this kind of research. The core of the HMI system focuses on the heart, both energetically and physically, as a vital source of innate intelligence. They found a critical link between the emotions and the heart, going beyond the idea that the heart is just a muscle pumping blood. The heart has its nervous system (McCraty & Childre, 2002; McCraty, 2006;

McCraty, 2015), and plays an important role in how we think and feel. Emotions are reflected in the patterns of our heart rhythms, and positive emotions help us maintain a coherent heart rhythm pattern, while negative emotions create incoherent patterns.

HMI has developed techniques that help to shift our rhythms from disordered to coherent, and those shifts translate into positive changes in our emotional states. We can neutralize the negative emotions when we connect with the power of our heart. The Quick Coherence° Technique is a wonderful way to create that heart coherence, shift our moods and attitudes, and to re-establish a more emotionally balanced and centered place. Here's the link to learn the technique: https://www.heartmath.com/quick-coherence-technique/. May you enjoy emotional health in these turbulent times.

Introducing Energy Medicine

Before exploring the value of energy medicine for renewal after having a baby, the next section describes how energy medicine affects the newborn in a specific way.

The Vivaxin Syndrome

As part of my training in energy medicine, I learned about a phenomenon called the Vivaxin Syndrome (Eden & Feinstein, class 2 Handout, 2012). Vivaxis is a term coined by Frances Nixon in Canada in the 1960s, and it refers to the energy that attaches a baby's energy field with the earth at the time of the birth. The theory explains that because there is an energy difference between the environment of the womb and the outside world, the body creates a magnetized field around the baby that acts like a force that bridges the transition from womb to the external world. To ensure the baby's safety, and protect it from shock, a meridian called Triple Warmer creates this magnetic field to serve as a protective shield for the first three months or the fourth trimester. It can save a baby's life by minimizing birth trauma. The Vivaxin field has polarities independent of the earth's magnetic field and is adapted to the baby's body moving with it rather than the earth. This magnetic field is designed to disintegrate early in the baby's life when it is no longer necessary, and if it does not dissolve after the first 3 months, a Vivaxin Syndrome can develop. When Triple Warmer detects stress, tension, or threats to the infant, it keeps the Vivaxin intact like a bubble of protection through childhood and into adulthood.

When someone has a Vivaxin Syndrome, their energies are weakened when they are facing in a particular direction: the direction in which the person was born, making them more vulnerable anytime they are facing in this specific direction. If there has been a traumatic or difficult birth, the Vivaxis becomes a potent force of protection that remains in place to accommodate the challenges presented by life on earth. The magnetic direction was set at birth, and when the person faces this direction later in life, it interferes with the body's other energies, rather than protecting them.

There are energetic ways of testing for and dissolving the syndrome, but that is beyond the scope of this book. I was fascinated to learn about this, after being a birth professional and parenting expert for decades. Without knowing that it had a name, I have observed this energy in young infants that came to my classes and groups over the years and noticed when it dissolved, and the baby became more engaged with the environment.

Daily Energy Medicine Can Help

The training that I had in Eden Energy Medicine has been an exciting development for me. It explains how the body utilizes energy for life, how our emotions affect and are affected by energy patterns, and how we connect to our environment by using energy. It is truly the way of the future. Energy medicine or healing is working with the subtle energies of the body and its electromagnetic field. In Eden Energy Medicine, there are nine systems that we work with, and they include meridians, chakras, radiant circuits, the aura, Celtic Weave, the basic grid, electrics, the 5 Rhythms, and Triple Warmer. Some of the basic principles of energy medicine are:

- ► energy wants to move, and it wants to do this in specific patterns,
- ► energy wants to cross over and can be seen by some as figure-8s all around the body,
- ► energy needs space to move, or it gets blocked and constricted,
- ► the way the body's energies flow, balance, and harmonize is reflected in the health of the body,
- ► all energies are interconnected, and therefore, we are affected by others and events in the environment,

► energy can form habits resistant to change, even when they are harmful, and

► energies can be repatterned.

The Daily Energy Routine (DER) is a set of exercises/movements that help you to restore the natural circulation and flow of energy throughout your body and the energy field surrounding it. During this postpartum time of low energy, doing the routine is an excellent way to recharge your batteries in less than 10 minutes. You can feel the difference in your energy flow when you start to do the routine on a regular basis. The exercises are tools to help you change your energy habits, some of which can develop from stress or illness; by reinstating an optimal flow, you can ease ordinary discomforts, acute and chronic illnesses, and the mental and emotional distress so common in the postpartum period.

You can foster an increased awareness of your body's energies and energetic needs and rebalance them by creating a dialogue with your body's energy systems. When your energies are humming, your baby is going to respond positively, since we know that the baby is enveloped within your aura, mentioned earlier in the section on the 40 days. You can take control of your energy flow and healing at a time when you may feel overwhelmed with new learning—an empowering experience when you can help yourself feel better. This leads to a stronger energetic core and a heightened sense of wellbeing, as you bring your energies into better integration, coherence, and flow.

When doing the DER, always breathe in through your nose and out through your mouth. The reason for this is it hooks up two meridians: the central meridian that goes up the front of the body, and the governing meridian that goes up the back and over the head. They meet at the back of the throat, so this breathing helps to connect them. Here is a link to Donna Eden's official version of the YouTube Daily Energy Routine that people enjoy following: https://www.youtube.com/watch?v=Di5Ua44iuXc (with some differences). Recently, I found another YouTube video of the DER by Prune Harris, another gifted Eden Energy Medicine practitioner, who has included the Neurolymphatic Reflex Points in her demonstration: https://youtu.be/nN2uq78Y2bE.

You will find in the section below that there are some parts of the DER that are self-explanatory in the words that are written. Other positions may not be so clear, so the photos can show you where on the body to touch or how the body should be positioned to get the full benefit.

Daily Energy Routine

The Daily Energy Routine starts with **4 Thumps**:

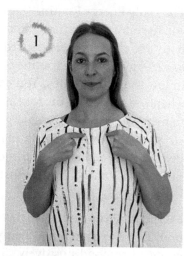

1. tapping on points under your eyes on the cheekbones (stomach meridian),

2. below your collarbone towards the center on the K27 points (kidney meridian) as shown in the image #1,

3. on the thymus at the sternum, and

4. on one of two sets of spleen points, either under the armpits #2 or a rib below the breasts in line with the nipples. #3

Tapping on these points is done for at least 15 seconds each. The **Cross Crawl** is like marching in place, touching one hand to the opposite knee, for about a minute, and getting the energies to cross over.

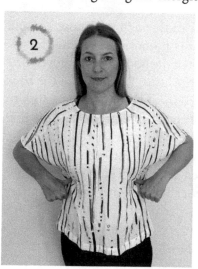

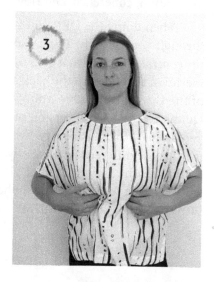

The next posture is called the **Wayne Cook Posture**, and it can be done in two ways: one sitting and an alternative in the standing position. These postures help when your energy is scrambled and involves crossing legs and arms, which can be seen in the #4 picture.

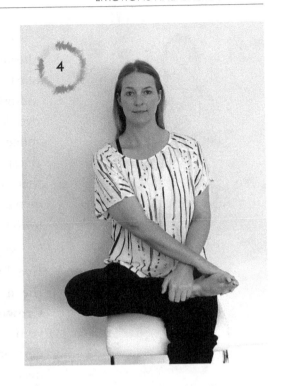

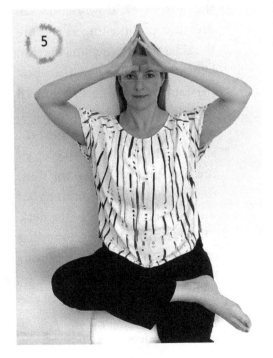

After doing five breaths on each side (in through the nose and out through the mouth), switch arms and legs to the other side, then steeple your fingertips, **#5** and place the thumbs on the third eye, just above the bridge of the nose, and take another five breaths while the thumbs move apart on the outbreath (although the model has her legs still crossed, you can sit normally during the steeple).

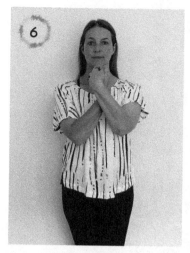

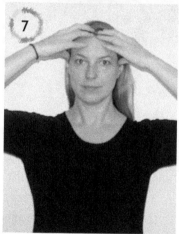

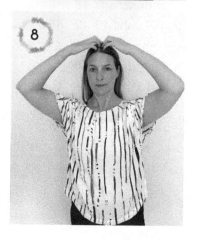

On this page we have the alternative standing position, #6. Starting with your arms extended in front, cross your arms and hands over, lace your fingers together, and rotate the clasped hands through the space between your arms, and then cross your ankles, so the same arm and leg are in front, and then switch sides.

Steeple the hands with the five breaths and this leads to the next movement, called the **Crown Pull**. With thumbs on your temples and rounded fingers at the center of your forehead (a little more rounded than the image) **#7**, slowly and with pressure, pull the fingers apart to the sides while stretching the skin beneath your fingers. Then repeat this starting at the hairline **#8** (here the fingers are well rounded) and pulling to the ears using pressure. Continue across the top of the head and pulling to the sides, the back of the head, working your way down to the base of the neck. Then, with your fingers pressing into both shoulders hold, pull your hands forward towards your front, and let them land in front of the chest, around your heart center, and take a deep breath.

After this, it's time to clear out the stagnant energy in your **Neurolymphatic Points**. The diagram shows where the points are and when you feel into them they might be tender, especially if they are clogged up. Massaging the points for about five seconds will help to clear them out.

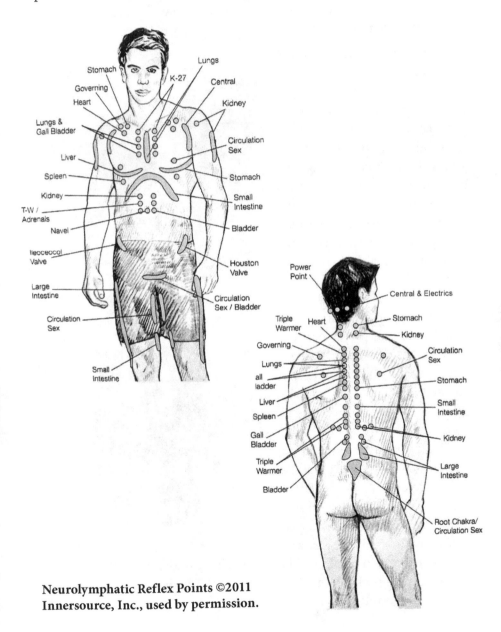

Neurolymphatic Reflex Points ©2011 Innersource, Inc., used by permission.

The **Zip-up and Lock** helps to protect you from negative energies while boosting confidence and is done by placing both hands on the pubic bone and pulling up along the front of the body up to the lower lip, and then complete the extension of your arms up and circle them around to the pubic bone again. Do this another time, and on the third round bring your fingers up to the lower lip and move your hands as if you were turning a key to lock in the Zip-up.

The next posture is the **Hook-up:** placing your middle finger of one hand on the third eye, and the other middle finger in your navel, and pull both fingers up. Hold for 15 to 30 seconds, or longer, if you want. **Connecting Heaven and Earth** activates spleen meridian for immune function, and also opens energies throughout the body, especially the joints. Starting with hands on the thighs and fingers spread, inhale and circle your arms out to the side, over your head and bring your hands in a prayer position in front of your heart. Exhale. While inhaling, stretch one arm up and the other down, with flat palms, and stretch the arms in both directions **#9**. Hold, and exhale, returning to prayer position. Switch arms and repeat the arms stretch in opposite directions. Do this twice for each side, and then with arms down, fold 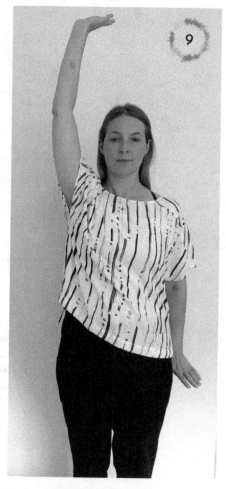 your body forward and over at the waist and take two breaths while you are bent over; each breath will bring you closer to the floor. Then, slowly roll your spine back up, making figure 8s with your arms as you return to a standing position.

The **Celtic Weave** exercise reinforces the Celtic Weave energy system, which forms figure-8 crossovers all over the aura, weaving the aura back together so it can protect you. Starting with hands on thighs, take a deep breath and then rub your hands together. Shake them off and feel the energy between your palms. Rub, shake off, and then place your palms close to your ears **#10** and breathe in and out. Inhale, bringing your elbows close together **#11**, and exhale, crossing your arms and swinging them out to the side, outstretched **#12**. Bending forward, cross and swing your arms out in front of your waist. Bend forward and repeat the movement in front of the knees, and then in front of the ankles. Bending your knees, turn your palms forward and scoop up the energy **#13** while returning to a stand with arms overhead, and let the energy rain down around you.

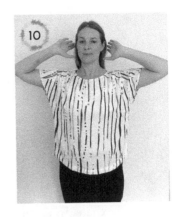

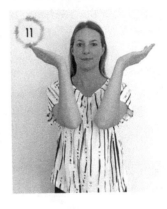

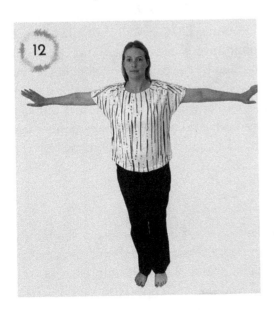

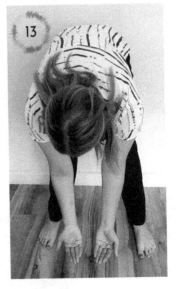

Finally, the last movement is **Heaven Rushing In**, which opens up support from "heaven." With feet shoulder width apart, rub your hands together and place your palms on your thighs, grounding the energy. Inhaling, circle your arms around in to prayer position, as you did in Connecting Heaven and Earth. Hold and exhale. Inhaling, reach both arms up overhead, opening your hands and heart to the

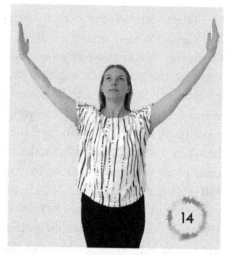

14

energy rushing at you from heaven #14. Exhale and hold this position for as long as you like, breathing normally. When ready, move your (overlapping) hands to your heart area, bringing heaven's energy with them. This place is called "heaven rushing in" and is a vortex that pulls the energy into your being. Breathe slowly and deeply and move your hands to any part of your body that might need some healing attention. Finish by bringing your hands back to the vortex.

Once you have done all these exercises, you will feel renewed. You can do this at the start of your day, or you can do what I do, and finish your day with the Daily Energy Routine. That way, all your energies are flowing and your systems are humming when you get into bed, even though you are bound to be woken up by the baby soon enough. Or you can choose any time of day that works best for you. You can also do this as a team with your partner, and both of you can benefit. I can't think of a better way to manage the common stresses of the fourth trimester than the Daily Energy Routine. I wish I had known about it when I was having my children.

►◄

As the fourth trimester ends, and integration is complete, the family emerges more connected and unified. Everyone's needs and insecurities were assuaged, and the love that was allowed to blossom enriches the bonds between everyone. Once again, there appears to be a horizon that extends beyond the cocoon of home, and activities in the world are resumed. Although it may have started earlier, mothers often find classes or groups with other mothers, which result in a new sense of community. Couples begin to go out alone again, using babysitters who offer a little respite from the 24/7 reality of parenting in the early stages. Life goes on in a new and expanded way.

The Mother of Hormones: Oxytocin

When we talk about hormones, we seem to lump them all together in some amorphous mass without any real understanding of what individual hormones do. We say things like "she's being hormonal" and "her hormones have got the best of her." Notice there aren't many references to men being hormonal. When I first started teaching childbirth preparation, we knew about oxytocin, prolactin, endorphins, estrogen, and progesterone, and the way in which they interacted during pregnancy, birth, and lactation. That was just the tip of the iceberg. Research over the last 30 years has expanded our awareness of a wide range of hormones and their impact on the body and the emotions, including for fathers.

In January 2015, Childbirth Connection published a noteworthy report on the *Hormonal Physiology of Childbearing: Evidence and Implications for Women, Babies, and Maternity Care*, written by Sarah Buckley, MD, a physician who has researched and practiced a gentle approach to pregnancy, birth, and parenting (www.ChildbirthConnection.org/HormonalPhysiology). This in-depth exploration presents the physiology of childbearing processes and how maternity-care practices can impede the flow of various hormones including oxytocin, prolactin, beta-endorphins, the stress hormones epinephrine/adrenaline, norepinephrine, and dopamine (collectively called the catecholamines), which will be discussed in Chapter 8. The report is a restorative for balancing out the medicalization of childbirth and presents the optimal possibility for what nature has intended when we observe and practice a physiological approach to the childbearing year, contrasted with how we connect with others, our social awareness, healing, and experience of closeness and intimacy.

Kerstin Uvnas Moberg wrote *the* book on oxytocin, *The Oxytocin Factor*, in 2003, five years after I finished teaching birth classes. How I would have loved to have had the knowledge in her book to share with my clients preparing for birth. This book has become a classic on the subject, and Uvnas Moberg is a sought-after expert and speaker who I've had the privilege of connecting with over lunch with colleagues, and more recently at a conference at which we were both presenting papers. Since its publication, research continues (including new volumes by Uvnas Moberg) to highlight how interference with oxytocin flow can have harmful effects on the mother, baby, and on a variety of natural behaviors. These maternal behaviors are being altered by the worldwide epidemic of inductions by synthetic oxytocin, prevalent in obstetric units throughout the industrialized world, with serious consequences in the lives of families after birth. I will return to this discussion later in the chapter.

Calm and Connection

Kerstin Uvnas Moberg describes oxytocin as part of the "calm-and-connection system," the polar opposite of the stress response (fight, flight, or freeze). The level of stress that people are living with has been ongoing for generations and dramatically increased in the 21st century, something that took a traumatic turn with the events on September 11, 2001. The fear that was generated by that day, and the political capital created around keeping people afraid, has had a powerful impact on the emotions of millions of people, reflected in the extraordinary increase in chronic diseases. Chronic inflammation, a fundamental part of the stress response that I will explore in Chapter 8, causes stress-related diseases, such as depression, diabetes, cancer, heart disease, and other cardiovascular illness. Chronic illness has overtaken acute illness in the use of medical resources.

The calm-and-connection system is the natural way that our bodies are designed to restore a healthy state of wellbeing and to counteract the effects of stress because oxytocin has anti-stress effects. The emotional tone of the calm-and-connection system is trust and curiosity, associated with friendliness in a way that predisposes us to see the world and others in a positive light. Oxytocin is the biological marker of the state of calm and connection. The balance of the stress response and the calm-and-connection system helps us sustain a healthy and optimal state of being.

Some of the contrasting attributes of the stress response and the calm-and-connection system are shown in the following table:

Stress Response	Calm-and-Connection Response
Stress	Rest
Confrontation	Peace
Pain	Pleasure
Loneliness	Companionship
Tension	Security
Commotion	Relaxation
Hunger	Satiety (feeling full)

Ideas borrowed from Uvnas Moberg, 2011; read the lists vertically as attributes of each system.

There will be a more detailed discussion of the stress response later.

Affiliation

Traditionally regarded as a female hormone because of its association with birth and lactation, we now know that oxytocin is produced by males and females, and can be activated through sensory stimuli, such as pleasant warmth and rhythmic touch. Sharing a meal with loved ones can have the effect of releasing oxytocin. Bodywork can also have this effect, and probably plays a significant part of the effectiveness of alternative forms of medicine or holistic healing. Because touch is an essential ingredient of bodywork, especially massage, it presents an opportunity for the release of oxytocin that restores calm and accelerates healing of all kinds. The benefits of massage for both recipient and practitioner create a state of wellbeing for both. All these social interactions are examples of affiliation with others, and how oxytocin influences our behaviors.

There are three prototypes of affiliation that are activated by oxytocin: parental bonds, pair bonds (romantic), and filial bonds (friendship). These are the connection part of the calm-and-connection system. Each of these bonds is partner-specific within the extended oxytocin system that provides the neurohormonal matrix for these different kinds of relationships. Affiliative bonds are defined as selective and enduring attachments with others. The bond that is created in early life with the parents, and especially the mother, will set the tone for future intimate relationships with others later in life. The anti-stress and anxiety-reducing effects of oxytocin support approach behaviors, rooted in the sense of safety, which facilitate bonding.

In pair and filial bonds, oxytocin may enhance social affiliation through the sense of wellbeing associated with close bonds, and the role of oxytocin in promoting health. Attachment partners shape each other's physiology through joint interactive behavior within a specific social context (Feldman, 2012). Similarly, parental oxytocin shapes the infant's emerging neuropeptide organization and its lifetime effects on social affiliation. The parents' early behavior and neuroendocrine response predict more reciprocal dialog and greater empathy between the next generation and their close friends.

The social context and individual differences moderate the central release of oxytocin, shaping which social behaviors and contexts trigger the release of endogenous oxytocin. Two different behavioral and motivational states are related to high levels of oxytocin: "tend and befriend," exemplified by relaxed parent-infant interactions that engender affiliative and nurturing motivations, and "tend and defend," which describes in-group vs. out-group interactions that are affiliative and defensive: trust and cooperation within the in-group, and defensive behavior toward the out-group. Oxytocin's key role in social bonding has short- and long-term effects. In the short run, it is a key component of pair bonds and bond formation between mother and offspring. The neural effects are likely to increase the probability of repeated, affiliative social interactions with particular individuals. In the long run, the social experience of childhood has long-term effects on the oxytocin system, impacting on mothering styles for females later in life. "Mothering styles, for example, alter an offspring's oxytocin gene receptor (OXR) expression, which then remains unchanged into adulthood" (Crockford et al., 2014, p. 2). To clarify how contextual variation and individual differences alter relationship dynamics, future research might experiment with administered (exogenous) oxytocin in healthy humans as they interact in natural contexts with known social partners.

Positive social behaviors and social bonding are highlighted by repeated physical contact, in which touch, warmth, and other sensory stimuli are involved in the release of oxytocin. Socially released oxytocin would include supportive social groups, and I have certainly experienced the phenomenon of being at events in which we could practically touch the oxytocin bubble we were all bathed in. When everyone is secreting oxytocin, it's contagious. That's the glow we leave with when we've been at a positive social bonding experience like a conference, or workshop, or training program.

The release of oxytocin is highly conditionable. By that, we mean that positive social experiences are stored as memories, which can reactivate physiological responses that reinforce physical benefits. An example would be a mother whose breast milk lets down when she hears another baby cry. Equally, and unfortunately, it can be conditioned negatively, which blocks the usual physiological response, and can interfere with breastfeeding. This is why, as I said in the introduction to this part, we need to involve loved ones in helping to keep the scales tipped in the positive direction so that oxytocin can flow and generate the health-promoting benefits that help the whole family to thrive.

Coordinating Function

One fundamental characteristic of oxytocin is its coordinating function, unique in physiology, which differentiates it from other substances in the body. Within the autonomic nervous system, the **hypothalamus** is the control center of the brain that regulates the functioning of internal organs, and it works very closely with the **pituitary gland**, where the hormonal control system is. Strong feelings, like anger and fear, have a powerful effect on the autonomic activities of the body, causing changes in heartbeat, breathing, and the redirection of blood flow to certain parts of the body as part of the stress response. Feelings and their physical responses are linked in powerful ways. Oxytocin, and its close cousin vasopressin (only two

which is not physiological and has the harmful effect of turning off oxytocin receptors. What this can do is stop maternal production by creating a (dose-dependent) decrease in natural oxytocin, and under-stimulation of related behaviors and functions.

The outcome of induced birth can involve breastfeeding difficulties since the effect on those receptor cells will make it hard for oxytocin to reach the alveoli in the breasts. One study demonstrated that the use of synthetic oxytocin was associated with 33 fewer days of breastfeeding (Erickson & Emeis, 2017). This is not common knowledge for women being coaxed into inductions and is not part of an informed-consent process. If women knew that induction could cause trouble with breastfeeding later, would they agree to the process? I wonder.

There are long-term effects on the endogenous oxytocin system, making it harder to trigger its release. Synthetic oxytocin also increases the risk of postpartum hemorrhage because it interferes with the normal pattern of the third stage (delivery of the placenta). Blood pressure and cortisol levels are elevated two days later when synthetic oxytocin has been used in labor, modifying the benefits of downregulating the stress response that comes with natural oxytocin flow and its anti-anxiety effect. Now let's see what other hormones are prevalent in the postnatal period.

CHAPTER 7

Prolactin and Other Reproductive Hormones

In the orchestra of ubiquitous postpartum hormones, prolactin—the mothering hormone[1] is the hallmark of breastfeeding, causing the breasts to produce milk at the end of pregnancy and after birth. Blood levels are high in the first weeks after birth, and frequent breastfeeding causes the creation of more prolactin receptors in the milk-producing cells of the breast (Behnke, 2003). The more receptors there are, the better the milk-making process will be, since prolactin will naturally decrease as the baby grows older and the high level of receptors means the production will continue efficiently down the road. Nursing your baby frequently in the first six weeks increases the likelihood of a plentiful supply of milk when the baby is 3 and 4 months old.

Prolactin, as its name suggests, is one of the lactation hormones and it works in synchrony with oxytocin. Levels of both these lactogenic hormones are highest in the first 10 days of breastfeeding and levels of prolactin rise and fall in proportion to the frequency, intensity, and duration of nipple stimulation/suckling. During pregnancy, when it is being manufactured by the placenta, there is a steady rise in prolactin levels (in conjunction with human-placental lactogen) causing the enlargement and activation of the mammary glands in preparation for milk production. Milk production increases as levels of progesterone decrease at the end of pregnancy.

After birth, prolactin is activated by the baby suckling, and once the placenta is delivered, the pituitary gland starts the job of secreting prolactin.

---

1   Some would say that is also oxytocin, which I think of as the love hormone because of its association with affiliative bonds.

The secretion of pituitary prolactin is regulated by the hypothalamus in a similar way to oxytocin, though they are secreted from different parts of the pituitary gland. Human-placental lactogen also helps to shape the brain for maternity, and after-birth prolactin continues to activate maternal behaviors, causing mothers to be more responsive to their babies, e.g., picking up their babies when they cry. It is prolactin that makes it hard to ignore a baby's cries, and we are hard-wired to connect with our babies because of prolactin's influence.

Lactation is maintained by the baby's sucking on the breast, promoting prolactin release that fills the breast with milk for the next feed. Males also produce prolactin, and both expectant fathers and new fathers have increased levels of prolactin concentrations in their bodies compared to men without partners. By spending intimate time carrying a baby and providing infant care, the hormonal impact on fathers will be similar, making them more responsive to their baby's cries.

A variety of other hormones can have an impact on prolactin production, increasing and decreasing the amount of prolactin that is released. The hormone dopamine, one of the catecholamines, plays a major role in reward-motivated behavior and is also produced by the hypothalamus. As a regulator of prolactin, the more dopamine there is, the less prolactin is released because of its role in the stress response, to be discussed in Chapter 8.

Estrogen is another regulator of prolactin, having the opposite effect of increasing the production and secretion of prolactin. My thinking about this has evolved over the years as more information has become available. Once believing that a decrease in estrogen production could lead to insufficient milk supply, it now seems that it's an increase in estrogen that causes this, but frequent nursing avoids this by suppressing estrogen. When estrogen is high, milk production plummets.

Like oxytocin, prolactin acts like an anti-stress hormone, helping the mother to stay calm through the challenging aspects of newborn mothering. Generally, breastfeeding mothers have lower levels of stress hormones. When working together with oxytocin, these hormones have a tranquilizing effect on the mother, and indirectly on the baby. When the baby absorbs prolactin, it aids fluid, sodium, potassium, and calcium transport. The biological half-life of prolactin is approximately half an hour, and this means that levels drop by 50% a half hour after feeding.

By comparison, oxytocin has a half-life of a few minutes (though recent research is adjusting this time frame). These are the biochemical facts that support frequent feeding in the early days after birth.

Prolactin Postpones Menstruation

Prolactin is known to suppress ovulation. Exclusive breastfeeding delays the return of menstruation, and it's called lactational amenorrhea (LAM). This happens because prolactin inhibits both gonadotropin-releasing hormone (GnRH), the hormone that allows eggs to develop and mature, and follicle-stimulating hormone (FSH), the hormone that triggers ovulation. In addition, prolactin also triggers the production of progesterone, which keeps the ovaries secreting progesterone. The length of time a woman goes without a period varies and can last for up to a year. My experience was that I started menstruating when my daughter was about 9 months old, and when my son was 8 months old (they were both breastfed for two years).

Although LAM is the most widely used birth control for women around the world, for Western women who use alternative feeding practices, it won't be. You will want to also be using some form of barrier method (condom, diaphragm, cervical cap) of contraception to minimize your fertility at this time. Many women end up pregnant again because they didn't use additional contraception. The hormonal suppression of ovulation and menstruation requires that no other form of food is given to the baby – neither formula nor solids, and also avoiding pacifiers. Exclusive breastfeeding both day and night provides that benefit, including night-time breastfeeding, but the introduction of other foods results in increased fertility and the possibility of conception. Nighttime feeding is important because prolactin peaks between the hours of 1:00 am to 6:00 am. For prolonged infertility, take advantage of those hours of high prolactin production during the night.

Levels of endorphins peak about 20 minutes into breastfeeding and are present in breast milk. Research shows that endorphin levels in breast milk at four days postpartum in mothers who have given birth vaginally are much higher than for mothers who had a cesarean (Zanardo et al., 2001). The extra dose of endorphins is believed to help the newborn cope with the stress of being born. During regular interactions between mother and baby, endorphins contribute to the pleasure of mutual dependency and reciprocal behaviors that nourish the connection between them, such as skin-to-skin contact and breastfeeding.

Hormonal Interactions and Imprinting

Endorphins also have a complex interaction with other hormones, and we still don't completely understand how the dynamics work. Endorphins are known to suppress the immune system, to ensure that a pregnant woman's body does not reject the unborn baby growing within her. We know that high levels of endorphins can inhibit the release of oxytocin, which allows a laboring woman to pace herself during birth, and could prevent premature birth too.

Babies secrete endorphins during labor from their pituitary gland and through the placenta and its membranes, so that levels in the placenta at birth are higher than those in the mother's bloodstream. Buckley raises the point that early cord clamping and cutting can deny the mother and baby the opioid molecules that are designed to promote bonding after birth. It also denies babies up to 30% of their blood causing anemia. There seems to be a reciprocal relationship between prolactin and endorphins, as elevated levels of prolactin also stimulate endorphin activity, reinforcing the rewards for intimate contact. The same is true for high levels of oxytocin, which can prevent opioid tolerance even in natural forms (as it does with narcotics) so that the rewards for maintaining contact remain high. One wonders, in these days of epidemic opioid addiction, if the addiction isn't compensating for the absence of oxytocin experiences in those who become addicted.

"Hormonal imprinting" takes place the first time a maturing receptor cell encounters its target hormone and sets the binding capacity of the receptor for life. Endorphins reward the baby for feeding, and the first episodes of suckling organize neural pathways in the newborn's brain, conditioning the baby to continue this pleasant activity. Therefore some breastfed babies experience confusion when given bottles because this creates an association of pleasure with both bottle teats and the mother's breast. Positive opiate bonding, internally and interactively, makes separation an upsetting experience, and for the baby, decreasing endorphin levels in the brain can be physically uncomfortable. Endorphin release is associated with mothering behaviors intrinsic to the reward system mentioned above, so the introduction of synthetic forms of opiates during birth can disrupt the maternal circuit.

Artificial forms of opiates, like narcotics and other drugs, can produce lifelong effects when they cause faulty imprinting at the start of life. Their consumption later in life can be seen as substitutes for close family connections. For some 30 years, research from the Karolinska Institute in Sweden has connected the use of analgesia in labor and addictive behaviors in the offspring of mothers given that form of pain relief (there are also associations between other obstetric interventions and self-destructive behaviors in the offspring, research led by Bertil Jacobson). When I first heard of this as a member of the Pre and Perinatal Psychology Association of North America (now called the Association for Prenatal and Perinatal Psychology and Health), the link between cause and effect had a mysterious feel to it. Now, the massive expansion of neuroscience has explained how this happens. The kinds of changes that occur in brain structure and function may not be revealed until the person becomes an adult.

The issues of hormonal imprinting are true for endorphins and the other hormones included in this chapter. Potent primary imprinting for the mother and baby is intended so that they can find and recognize each other in the hours and days after birth, probably a remnant of our mammalian roots. High oxytocin levels familiarize a mother with the unique odor of her newborn infant, called olfactory recognition, so that she prefers her own baby's smell over others. Babies are similarly imprinted to their mothers, and at birth are already imprinted to the smell of the amniotic fluid. This "odor imprint" helps newborns find their way to the mother's nipple during the breast crawl (which is described in more detail in the breastfeeding part of this book) from the abdomen to the breast, which has a similar but slightly different scent. In the days following birth, the infant is comforted by these imprints to odor.

Estrogen and Progesterone

These two hormones are the structure on which a woman's reproductive life is organized and play their most exalted roles during pregnancy. However, during the postnatal period, both hormones are in their nadir, at the lowest levels in a woman's experience, once the expulsion of the placenta during the third stage of labor is complete. Unlike the other hormones that have a prominent role to play during this time, these two hormones are being presented together as they often work synergistically. This means that the combined effect of both hormones acting together is greater than the sum of their individual effects. These two sex hormones are steroids, and they play out their roles during the menstrual cycle monthly until pregnancy occurs. Estrogen causes the physiological changes in a female body during puberty, initiating the menstrual cycle.

There are three types of estrogen: 1) estrone, a relatively inactive form made in fat tissue, 2) estradiol, made in the ovaries and responsible for the physical changes in the body, and 3) estriol, the main player during pregnancy. As the primary hormone for ovulation, it signals the time when fertilization is likely to take place. Progesterone, the hormone of progestation, is the essential ingredient for pregnancy to happen; it enlarges the endometrium, the lining of the uterus, with blood and nutrients for the implantation of a fertilized egg cell. Low levels of progesterone are a sign of probable miscarriage because there isn't enough juice for the endometrium to nourish the embryo or to keep the pregnancy going. Once pregnancy occurs, it is the placenta that will be producing estrogen and progesterone for the duration.

During pregnancy, estrogen controls the ripening of the cervix in preparation for birth, and it increases uterine receptors for oxytocin, which will cause the uterus to contract. Estriol levels increase by more than 1,000 times and surge in the moments leading up to the onset of labor. With the delivery of the placenta, the woman's source of estrogen plummets and the estrogen level drops to 10% of the prenatal value within three hours postpartum. It reaches the lowest level around day seven postpartum, and this is the equivalent to the level of estrogen in postmenopausal women.

During pregnancy, progesterone has a relaxing effect on the uterus that prevents premature contractions and birth and keeps lactation in check before the delivery of the baby. Progesterone levels are 10 to 18 times higher than non-pregnant levels. Progesterone levels also plummet after birth and are undetectable by 72 hours after delivery, and will only be re-established when the mother has her first menstrual cycle. The dramatic drop in these hormone levels at delivery marks the onset of milk production, the hormonal trigger for lactation to begin. Low estrogen causes vaginal tissue to remain thin after birth, causing dryness that is best managed with lubricating ointments. Lower libido (interest in sex) is another aspect of diminished estrogen levels. The significance of these hormones during the postnatal period has more to do with their deficit and the impact it has on women's moods.

Impact of Low Levels of Sex Hormones

Menopause, or more accurately perimenopause, is sometimes seen as an estrogen-deficiency issue and other theories see it as an issue of "estrogen dominance." There are similar views about estrogen dominance in the postnatal period. What this means is that even though both hormones drop dramatically, estrogen levels are still present at 10% compared to progesterone, and this is called "unopposed estrogen." One wonders if this has something to do with the "baby blues," which seems to coincide with the disappearance of progesterone around 72 hours postpartum. Estrogen dominance can lead to thyroid dysfunction, because estrogen causes the liver to produce a substance that binds thyroid hormone, making it unavailable as energy for the cells of the body.

Another issue is adrenal fatigue, where estrogen has a similar effect of increasing a cortisol-binding substance, causing a serious decrease in free cortisol available to cells, and interfering with the release of cortisol from the adrenal cortex. Since cortisol is one of the hormones that is derived from progesterone (and cholesterol), progesterone's decline interferes with cortisol production. Any of the circumstances—adrenal-cortex inhibition, limited cortisol production, or binding of cortisol—can lead to adrenal fatigue, and this, in turn, can interfere with bonding. Mothers with appropriate levels of cortisol are more responsive to their babies, especially their baby's smell, which is associated with a stronger mother/infant bond.

Still, the more popular theory is estrogen deficiency after birth. Estrogen is involved in the production of serotonin, a neurotransmitter in

Catecholamines activate the sympathetic nervous system (SNS), which increases blood pressure, heart rate, breathing, and moves blood flow away from organs and out to the muscles of our extremities in preparation for fleeing as fast as possible. When the crisis is over, the reverse actions are activated by the parasympathetic nervous system (PNS), where norepinephrine rules. This downregulates the system and restores the state of balance (homeostasis) important for good health, making us more receptive to the calm-and-connection system.

The sympathetic and parasympathetic nervous systems are part of the autonomic nervous system, which controls the visceral functions of the body, and operates below the level of conscious control, compared to the central nervous system in which we control our actions and responses. The parasympathetic nervous system takes care of background operations, such as heart/lungs and digestion, and the sympathetic nervous system initiates the stress response, as well as procreative functions and strategies. There are now approaches for accessing the autonomic nervous system on a more conscious level, taking the autonomic nervous system off autopilot, such as biofeedback, neurofeedback (for brain regulation), and deep conscious breathing.

Years ago, I was trained to believe that adrenaline and oxytocin are antagonists – the presence of adrenaline has a diminishing effect on oxytocin. What I have learned since is that it is corticotropin-releasing hormone (CRH, or corticotropin-releasing factor, CRF), part of the HPA axis, that is the culprit. This antagonism plays out during birth when high levels of adrenaline's beta cells block oxytocin release, slowing down labor, and decreasing blood flow to the uterus and placenta, and eventually to the baby. The impact is longer labor and possible fetal distress due to the reduction in oxygenated blood flow to the unborn baby. However, at the moment of delivery, the alpha cells of norepinephrine stimulate the fetus-ejection reflex that pushes the baby out with the strong contractions they produce.

It is the ratio of adrenaline to norepinephrine that's important, as both these types of receptors are sensitive to adrenaline in the uterus. The level of these catecholamines normally drops significantly after the birth, but the risk of postpartum hemorrhage increases when high levels of catecholamines constrict oxytocin flow, which keeps the uterus contracting after the baby is born.

Adrenaline release is contagious, and during birth, it's essential to keep levels of adrenaline low in the laboring woman, as well as anyone who surrounds her. Whether that is her partner, mother, nurse, midwife, doctor, or anyone else that is generating catecholamine release, emotional contagion will impede the flow of oxytocin. Dr. Michel Odent believes the authentic midwife sits in the corner and knits while a woman is in labor because this repetitive action keeps adrenaline at a minimum, and it allows the mother to get on with giving birth spontaneously and instinctively. He also calls the neocortex of the brain a human handicap for birthing women because overthinking takes us out of our right mind for birth.

Postpartum Effects of Catecholamines

So, what does this mean for mothers in the postpartum period? When a new mother is stressed and produces elevated catecholamines, this can interfere with oxytocin reaching the breasts and inhibit the secretion of milk. We know that these hormones, particularly CRH, put a brake on oxytocin flow, and the let-down or milk-ejection reflex will be impacted. Both CRH and oxytocin come from the paraventricular nucleus of the hypothalamus.

The anti-stress effects that occur with each breastfeeding, such as the lowering of blood pressure and cortisol levels, are lost. Reviewing how oxytocin commands the calm-and-connection system that offsets the stress response, we can lose the anti-stress benefits of oxytocin beyond the breastfeeding experience, such as with positive social interactions and emotions. Oxytocin has so many health-promoting effects that we don't want to mess with it during this tumultuous time. Oxytocin is easily conditioned to psychological states, both positive and negative, and we benefit from the regulatory effects it provides for long-term positive life experiences.

The fight/flight/freeze response has diverse effects on the body. Activation of the sympathetic nervous system increases cardiac output and constriction in blood vessels, with additional effects on the kidneys, the digestive system, metabolism, the skin, and a rise in blood pressure. Corticotrophin-releasing factor (CRF) and vasopressin induce behavior changes, such as fear and aggression during a defensive reaction, and stimulate the release of adrenocorticotrophic hormone (ACTH) and cortisol. None of these physiological states are conducive to a calm-and-connected experience between mother and baby, or between parents, and will likely create a great deal of tension instead. When a newborn doesn't receive dependable oxytocin-producing responsive care, this raises levels of the stress hormone, cortisol. Studies have shown that chronic cortisol elevations in infants, and the corresponding hormonal and functional adaptations that occur, are associated with enduring brain changes that lead to heightened reactions to stress throughout life.

On the other hand, when oxytocin flows freely, it fosters the connection between mother and baby and between parents. As part of the protection and care of your baby, you not only give milk, but you transmit warmth to the baby as the blood vessels around the mammary glands dilate. You are both giving and receiving, since the baby's suckling, touching, and warmth activate your milk-ejection reflex. Both momentary and long-term relaxation (anti-stress) effects are induced, with a corresponding downregulation in the sympathetic response, and lowering blood pressure. An enhanced vagal-nerve tone, part of the shift from sympathetic to parasympathetic nervous response, aids the secretion of digestive hormones. Long-term adaptations for lactating women include more receptivity toward social interactions and calmness, the antithesis of the stress response.

Hypothalamic-Pituitary-Adrenal Axis

In a moment I'm going to discuss cortisol and its impact on the body. To fully understand how cortisol works, we need to have a look at the hypothalamic-pituitary-adrenal axis (HPA) and how this complex system of feedback interactions affects the organs involved: the hypothalamus, pituitary gland, adrenal glands, and beyond. The HPA axis controls reactions to stress, regulates a variety of body processes, and is the mechanism for interactions between glands, hormones, and parts of the brain. This simplified diagram (next page) shows how this plays out in the secretion of cortisol released by the adrenal gland for the general population.

Normally, there is a negative feedback loop so that high levels of cortisol will start downregulating the production of CRH. During pregnancy, this is different, and there is positive feedback on the placental production of CRH. The fetal adrenal gland is also producing cortisol in the last weeks of pregnancy, believed to be a sign of maturation of the fetal organs and related to the timing of birth. Despite high levels of all the hormones, the

HPA reactivity to stress is diminished in late pregnancy. Cortisol levels will return to normal within a couple of days after birth, and with breastfeeding women, the sympathetic tone and response to stress are lower after birth. Oxytocin is believed to have this positive influence on the HPA stress response during the postpartum period.

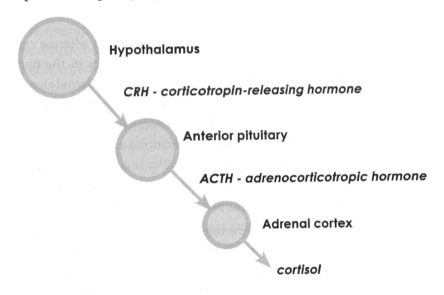

Hypothalamus

CRH - corticotropin-releasing hormone

Anterior pituitary

ACTH - adrenocorticotropic hormone

Adrenal cortex

cortisol

Similar to how low sex hormones are studied in relation to postpartum depression, cortisol levels are also being researched as a factor in postnatal psychological disturbances. There are correlations between high cortisol reactivity and heightened emotional reactions to psychosocial stress during pregnancy, and the incidence of postpartum depression in healthy women. Studies are testing how predictive this is for the probability of depression within weeks after birth.

For the general population, cortisol is sometimes called "the depression hormone," since it tends to show up when depressive symptoms are present, particularly for stress-induced clinical depression. In postpartum women with depression, there are elevated levels of cortisol in the blood. At the moment, there are inconsistent findings in the research (Meinlschmidt et al., 2010; Nierop et al., 2006) that has been done, but I would anticipate that in the future, the correlations will generate a more causal connection between higher reactivity during pregnancy and the experience of postpartum depression after birth. If so, there will be ways to treat women at risk to

the fetus marinates in stress hormones in the womb that influence those set points. This can be offset by consistent regular body contact with parents producing higher levels of oxytocin to lessen the stress response in the baby.

Oxytocin will regulate the permanent organization of the stress-handling part of the baby's brain, and this relates to how secure or insecure the person becomes later in life. I describe this in more detail in the Bonding and Attachment Part 4. As you can see, it can be a delicate balancing act to sustain enough cortisol for the positive effects and yet not produce an excess that causes the negative effects.

Inflammatory-Response System (IRS)

When catecholamines are activated, and the HPA axis is stimulated, this leads to the inflammatory-response system causing inflammation in the body. As mentioned above, I explain a new paradigm for what happens during perinatal depression (and other mood disorders) that involves the inflammatory response as the main risk factor, in *The Adverse Aftermath of Birth*. But inflammation is not just a marker for perinatal mood and anxiety disorders; it's a key factor in the stress response too (Kendall-Tackett, 2007).

The inflammatory response (inflammation) occurs when the body's tissues are injured by bacteria, trauma, toxins, heat, or any other cause, as a defense mechanism that evolved in higher organisms to protect them from infection and injury. The damaged cells release chemicals that cause blood vessels to leak fluid into the tissues, causing swelling. This helps isolate the foreign substance from further contact with body tissues. Inflammation works to localize and eliminate the injurious agent and to remove damaged tissue components so that the body can begin to heal. There are two types of inflammation: *acute* and *chronic* (sometimes called systemic) inflammation. Examples of acute inflammation would be a skin abrasion, an infected ingrown nail, a sprained ankle, acute bronchitis, a sore throat, tonsillitis, or appendicitis.

Chronic inflammation is long-term and occurs in "wear and tear" conditions, including osteoarthritis, autoimmune diseases (such as lupus and rheumatoid arthritis), allergies, asthma, and inflammatory bowel diseases (such as Crohn's disease). Probably the most well-known conditions that develop after years of inflammation are cardiovascular disease, cancer, diabetes, and depression.

The inflammatory response is an essential part of the immune system, and it is nonspecific and responds to various types of potential threats. That includes invasions by bacterial or viral infections, or damage to tissues like a sprained ankle, where connective tissues and muscles are torn. This tissue damage causes the release of inflammatory molecules that begin the inflammatory process, called cytokines. Cytokines are the key markers of inflammation, and they regulate the immune response, helping the body to fight infection and heal wounds by activating an inflammatory response. They cause small blood vessels, arterioles, to dilate and become leakier, bringing more blood into the area. Some cytokines attract white blood cells, neutrophils, and the leaky arterioles facilitate their movement out of the blood vessels and into the tissues where they can start fighting infection and repairing tissue damage. As leaky blood vessels allow cells out, they also leak fluid too, causing redness and swelling. Increased swelling causes pain as neighboring tissues are squeezed, triggering pain and pressure receptors.

Cytokines called pyrogens are also released to raise the temperature of the affected area. Sometimes, your entire body temperature may go up, and you may develop a fever, depending on the severity of the infection or injury. The "cardinal" signs of inflammation are four types of response that use Latin words to describe them: *calor* (heat), *dolor* (pain), *rubor* (redness), and *tumor* (swelling). These signs of inflammation were first described by physicians over 2000 years ago, and are still used to identify an acute inflammatory response.

Using the example of perinatal depression, one thing that happens when there is inflammation is the brain doesn't function in the way it is meant to. Research has demonstrated that physical and psychological stressors increase inflammation in the body, making inflammation a risk factor that underlies all the others. It also explains why psychosocial, behavioral, and physical risk factors (read: stressors) increase the risk of depression, considering women's levels of proinflammatory cytokines increase significantly in the third trimester of pregnancy. Some women are more vulnerable to the effects of inflammation than others, and those who have experienced premenstrual tension, a response to inflammation, are more susceptible to postpartum depression. Since new motherhood is fraught with stressors that can cause proinflammatory cytokines to rise, such as sleep deprivation, postpartum pain, and trauma, the goal would be to reduce maternal stress and inflammation for the prevention and treatment of perinatal depression (Kendall-Tackett, 2007). Stress management can be a new approach to perinatal mood and anxiety disorders.

Inflammation influences levels of hormones, such as serotonin and the catecholamines that we talked about earlier in this chapter, as well as the HPA axis, which (as we discussed) controls cortisol levels. Inflammation normally triggers the HPA axis to release cortisol and other inflammatory substances, such as C-reactive protein, and depression generates abnormalities, such as immune dysfunction and the down-regulation of the HPA axis, so that cortisol, normally an *anti-inflammatory hormone*, is not utilized effectively.

Depressed people can have 40% to 50% higher levels of inflammation than non-depressed people. There is a bidirectional relationship between inflammation and depression: inflammation increases the risk of depression, and depression increases inflammation. The nearly universal experience of sleep disruption and fatigue in the postpartum period is another cause of inflammation, which also has a bidirectional interaction: sleep disturbance increases cytokines and cytokines increase sleep disturbance (Kendall-Tackett et al., 2011). Pain and trauma are other risk factors for inflammation and depression, and PTSD, which is a dysregulation of the normal stress response, can reduce the pain threshold in women. Since cortisol's role is to inhibit the inflammatory response system, there is increased cytokine activity in people with PTSD. Stress and depression both augment the production of proinflammatory cytokines, which can lead to age-related chronic diseases later in life (Kendall-Tackett, 2007; 2009).

There is so much new data on the stress response that our knowledge keeps growing in exponential ways. That's been true since I first started to write about it several years ago, when I had a much less nuanced understanding. I hope this has been helpful to you in understanding what's happening when you feel stressed in the early days and weeks after your baby is born, and that you feel you have tools to manage it, which you'll find in Chapter 10. Next, we'll explore how fathers' hormones are helping them adapt to new parenthood too.

CHAPTER 9

Fathers and Hormones

One of the most exciting developments in the last decade is the discovery that fathers go through natural hormonal changes, along with their pregnant partners, that shape them into devoted dads.[2] We know that when the father is cohabiting with his mate, his oxytocin levels rise toward the end of her pregnancy. After birth, when the father spends significant amounts of time in contact with his baby, oxytocin helps to keep him engaged in the ongoing care of his infant. Nature provides fathers with the biological incentive to remain a dedicated and satisfied part of the family through his involvement with his baby. Oxytocin also increases his interest in being physically close to the mother, and not in a sexual way. Are the same things true for same-sex partners? I wonder...

Vasopressin, the hormone that controls blood pressure and fluid balance in the body, is active in the bonding process for the mother and baby, with a larger role to play in the father. This hormone reorganizes the brain for paternal behaviors when he is living with his pregnant partner, causing him to feel more dedicated to her. Vasopressin is released in response to closeness and touch (thanks to its association with oxytocin), which promotes bonding with the mother and with his baby, and inspires his desire to be part of this family. Called the "monogamy hormone," it has a tempering effect on his sexual drive, which is so useful when sex goes on to the backburner in the postpartum period. Vasopressin also reduces aggression, making him more rational, and prompts his paternal role for providing stability and vigilance. This promotes the father's protective instincts for his mate and child.

---

2   This chapter talks about the effect of hormones on the father based on recent research. I have not come across research that says whether the same thing would happen for a same-sex partner, but we cannot preclude that happening.

CHAPTER 10

Energy Medicine for Balancing Stress Hormones

To **simplify** your experience of the hormonal roller coaster during the early postpartum period, here are some energy techniques that can help control the antagonistic hormones of the stress response: catecholamines and cortisol. In the section on the fourth trimester, I introduced Triple Warmer (TW) as the creator of the Vivaxis when a baby is born. A special meridian that also functions as a radiant circuit, TW is responsible for keeping us alive and is intimately involved with the adrenal glands, where it governs the fight/flight/freeze response. TW has not adapted to the kinds of stress common in the 21st century, and it is still operating like there is a saber-toothed tiger about to pounce. If TW assesses a threat to the organism, it can borrow energy from other meridians for its survival. In stress-prone cultures, Triple Warmer is on alert most of the time, keeping it in a state of overdrive.

Meridians, or energy pathways, sit on a flow wheel where each one has a polar opposite, and the meridian that sits across from Triple Warmer is Spleen, responsible for metabolizing everything that we take in (food, chemicals, and emotional stressors). The relationship between TW and Spleen is unique because Triple Warmer is always taking energy from Spleen, so that TW is nearly always overenergized, and Spleen is almost always depleted. TW and Spleen meridians govern the immune system and each has a different but complementary role. A weak spleen means we are not able to adequately metabolize, integrate, or repel harmful input, and this can jeopardize our well-being. A chronically weakened Spleen meridian can lead to metabolic, chemical, and hormonal problems.

Triple Warmer governs and is governed by the hypothalamus, the control center of the brain that works so closely with the pituitary gland, the hormonal control center. Therefore, it will have a strong presence during the postpartum period, acting like a commander-in-chief focusing on danger and threat. It is also the keeper of habits, both positive and negative, and when we want to make adjustments of any kind, we need to enlist TW as an ally, or it will resist all attempts to change. When TW is out of balance, it can cause physical illnesses, such as adrenal exhaustion, digestive problems, and thyroid conditions. It also can cause psychological problems, including addictions, mood swings, and sleep issues, to name just a few. The objective is to keep it in balance with Spleen and other meridians, because when balanced, TW can promote feelings of safety, and warm and balanced social connections. Our feelings of joy, forgiveness, and gratitude positively influence it. Because it is so responsive to our thoughts and beliefs, for better or worse, it's important to be aware of its influence in our lives and to use techniques that keep it in balance.

Triple Warmer Smoothie

If you have ever smoothed your hair behind your ears, without realizing it you are calming down Triple Warmer. The meridian travels up the arm, neck, and around the ear to finish just beyond the temple close to the eyebrow. The action of tucking hair behind the ears is calming the energy in the meridian. This exercise is an intentional smoothing of the energy that extends the movement further. Rest your face in your hands, with your palms at the chin and fingers at the temples and hold for two breaths. While inhaling, move your fingers 2 to 3", smoothing the skin around the temples to above the ears. Exhaling, circle your fingers around your ears, press down the sides of your neck, and hang your hands on the back of your shoulders, pressing your fingers in. Stay like this for two deep breaths, and then drag the fingers with pressure forward over the shoulders and let your hands come together at the center of your chest at the heart. Take a deep breath to finish.

Tapping the TW "Fear Point"

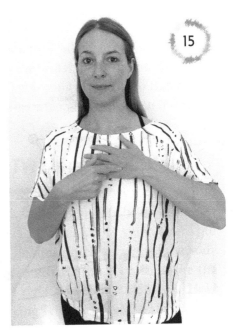

(#15) Place your left hand over the heart and tap 10 times on the point on the back of the hand between the ring and little fingers, just below the knuckles. Pause and take a deep breath. Tap another 30 times on this spot, or you can tap using four fingers along the entire ridge below the knuckle. If you are still feeling fearful, you can tap on the other hand the same way. For those of you that are familiar with energy psychology (see below), this is called the "gamut" point.

Calming TW Neurovascular Points

When we become stressed, blood rushes away from the forebrain and into the limbs to support the fight-or-flight response. The autonomic nervous system needs to react instantly, and our thinking brain is relatively slow and less effective. However, the stresses that we encounter today require us to be able to think clearly, and the main Neurovascular (NV) reflex points allow us to help the body learn to meet stress with a functioning forebrain. When we hold these points on our forehead, it pulls the blood flow back up to the brain, helping our clarity of thought and restoring our center emotionally. By holding the NV points, we can reprogram our responses to stress in a way that counteracts the "emergency response loop," and trains the primitive brain that the crisis is not a real danger. We are helping the brain to evolve how it responds to stress in a more balanced way. Most of the NV points are around the head, and TW Neurovascular points are at the temples and in the V of the throat, right above the collarbone. Make a three-finger notch with your right hand by bringing your thumb, index, and middle fingers together, and place it in the V above your clavicle. Place your left hand flat across the left side of your head, with fingers flat on the temples. Take three to five slow, deep breaths. Change hands and do the same on the other side.

These energy medicine/psychology tools can help you navigate some of the hormonal turbulence with some equanimity that will benefit you, your partner, and your baby. In the next section on breastfeeding, I want to share a wealth of information about this wonderful way of feeding our babies the perfect food for growth and development.

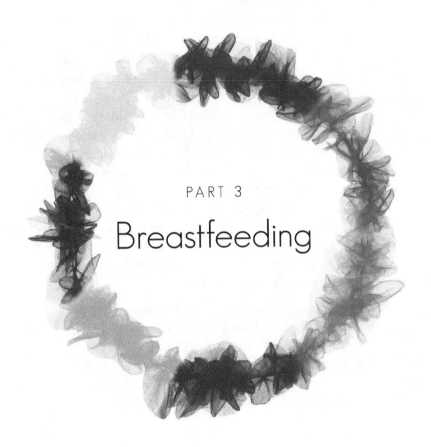

PART 3

Breastfeeding

PART 3 INTRODUCTION

The next few chapters focus completely on breast-feeding. My goal is to help mothers have a positive breastfeeding experience. I also want to acknowledge the heartbreaking reality of those mothers who tried to breastfeed and weren't able to do so, despite all their best efforts. They often have a negative reaction to articles and blogs about breastfeeding that can trigger some defensiveness about their own experiences. I've observed some confrontational threads on Facebook and other social media between breastfeeding advo-cates and those who couldn't do it and feel judged for not succeeding. They carry a sense of failure about the capacity to nurse a baby, even though we know that lack of support and help is what often causes premature weaning. It is not an individual problem; it's a societal problem when women are given so much contradictory information from different profession-als, or those same professionals are too busy to assist. It also is a public health problem.

Some women choose not to breastfeed, and they make this choice for many different personal reasons. I've had clients who had wonderful natural childbirths but opted to formula-feed. I'm not one to insist that women breastfeed, especially as there are so many barriers to being able to do it successfully.

For those unable to breastfeed and those who choose formula-feeding, more information on effective resources for this choice can be found here:

www.fearlessformulafeeder.com
www.babycenter.com
www.babycentre.co.uk

CHAPTER 11

Body Awareness
for Breastfeeding

In Part 2, we examined the various hormones that are governing the experience of new motherhood and their interactions. In this part, we will take a look at how to make the most of breastfeeding, because it has become such a complicated matter that we need to *simplify* the whole experience. Like birth, also a "complicated" experience these days, breastfeeding will flow if we don't interfere with it; and when I say interference, I am talking about mindsets that get in the way, as well as behaviors that can be counterproductive. There is an art to nursing your baby, and I want to support this for new mothers.

The Physiology of Breastfeeding

I wonder how many science classes these days provide information about lactation or breastfeeding. It seems the curriculum is averse to mentioning breasts, with all their sexual connotations. A recent Google search on whether millennials have been taught about breastfeeding showed results that recommend that this is taught in elementary schools, but no examples of it being taught. One study in Brazil examined science textbooks and found no themed curriculum on breastfeeding and suggested ways of integrating concepts into the textbooks (Galvao & Silva, 2013). There's a big move in the UK to teach breastfeeding in schools because of its very low breastfeeding rate. I like to think things have changed since my youth, but so far, I don't know that this subject is being taught in schools. So, let's fill in the gaps.

Prolactin is responsible for the production of milk and colostrum during pregnancy. It stimulates the growth of the alveoli, or milk-producing

CHAPTER 12

The Practicalities of Breastfeeding

Practical Aspects of Breastfeeding

Here's where we get into the nitty-gritty of breastfeeding. Women feel the let-down reflex in a variety of ways. Some women experience a tingling sensation. For others, the nipple becomes erect. Others feel twinges, and for some, it feels like a burning sensation. It can be felt high up in the glands of the breast, at the tip of the nipple, or around the breast. Some women are unaware of the let-down reflex at all, and often, it is with subsequent babies that it becomes more noticeable. There is a wide range of personal experiences with how the milk lets down, so it is good not to expect it to be a certain way.

Because it is the baby's sucking that causes the oxytocin to flow, and the milk-secreting cells to squeeze the milk into the ducts, continued sucking draws the milk out to the baby and stimulates the milk-ejection reflex. For the first 10 minutes, oxytocin is released in a pulsatile rhythm. When the baby is latched well, with as much of the areola in the baby's mouth as possible, then the milk continues to flow comfortably. Some women with large areolas might not get all of the areola into the baby's mouth, and the baby is still latched on well, so the important thing is to have an asymmetrical latch. Touching the top lip with the nipple, wait for the mouth to open (or gape), and then bring the baby in slightly off-centered to the nipple, so the chin is resting on the breast while he or she nurses. The head will be tilted back supported by the mother's hand pressing into the shoulders to prevent the chin from curling inward. Here's a link to a video created by Dr. Jack Newman (2011), a Canadian pediatrician-advocate for breastfeeding: https://youtu.be/NO5ZDKynaD0.

If babies only have the nipple in their mouths and are allowed to suck this way, this will lead to sore nipples, and the answer is to start again. A lot of women feel the suction all around the breast when the baby is latched. It is the suction in the baby's mouth that keeps the nipple in place, and it is the tongue and the jaws that draw the milk out. Breaking the suction is very important when taking the baby off the breast because the vacuum that is created by the baby's mouth is so strong. Sometimes babies will let go of the breast naturally and detach, but if that does not happen, then breaking the suction with the little finger is essential because once babies are latched on properly, they will not let go. Push your little finger (pinky) into the corner of the baby's mouth, and when a click is heard, indicating the suction has released, then the baby can be moved away from that breast. If the suction is not broken, the baby will pull the nipple out, which is another way to cause sore nipples.

Supply and Demand

Breast milk is produced according to the law of supply and demand. It is very simple; the more that is removed from the breasts, the more the body is going to produce. It is an exquisite rhythm created by nature to guarantee the flow that the baby needs. Using a quantitative approach, if a certain number of ounces are sucked out of the breast by the baby, then the same amount will be produced. As the baby grows over the first five weeks, it will need more ounces, so it will nurse more frequently until it removes a higher quantity, and then the body will get to work producing those extra ounces. After five weeks, the quantity remains stable for the duration of breastfeeding. You supply as much milk as the baby needs, providing you do not get caught up in the various ways that this rhythm can be inhibited.

Some babies are quick feeders but still get all they need. My son Jasper was one of those. He only ever took 10 minutes for a feeding, being extremely efficient in transferring milk. In the early days, I wondered if he was getting enough milk because of his brief feeds. So, I brought him to the pediatrician at a month just to check. This baby, who started life weighing 10 lbs. 4 oz., weighed 13 lbs. 14 oz. at 1 month. I stopped worrying. Equally, some babies take a long time to finish a feeding, taking their time at the breast, like two of my other children did. We need to be cautious not to create any false expectation about how long it should take because babies are unique and will do their own thing.

When the time comes that the mother/baby is ready to wean, the process works in reverse. If you want to cut out one feeding of X ounces, your body will adjust to producing X ounces less over the course of the day. Your body makes these adjustments over the weeks and months that you are weaning until the point where little or no breast milk is being produced because none is being withdrawn. This is another little miracle of breastfeeding to be admired. Some mothers continue to produce a small amount of milk, even when they have finished nursing. The size of the mother's breasts has nothing to do with the ability to produce milk. A woman with small breasts can produce as much milk as a woman with large breasts because the production happens in the milk-making cells, not in the fat tissue of the breasts. In most cases, regardless of the size of a woman's breasts, she can produce as much milk as her baby needs.

Growth Spurts

And then there are growth spurts. Like many other things in life, some babies have growth spurts on a two-week, four-week, and two-month rhythm, and other babies have a three-week, six-week, and three-month rhythm. This is not set in stone, and babies will find their way in having growth spurts. You won't know which one applies until your baby suddenly wants to nurse all the time after things have settled down into a nice "routine." There may be a 48-hour period (approximately) when all you seem to be doing is feeding the baby at the breast, and everything else seems to go by the wayside.

The best thing to do is to go with it because it will come to an end and go back to "normal," and a new routine will establish itself. However, at the end of the growth spurt, you will be producing enough milk to satisfy the baby at a higher level of production. This is an example of how the law of supply and demand is working—when the baby needs more ounces of milk, it nurses more frequently, and your body adjusts by producing those extra ounces of milk to replace what was removed. Once the higher level is established, the frequency of feedings will return to a rate similar to before the growth spurt happened.

resolve this temporary, daily phenomenon. It's a good idea to plan for the baby needing to nurse more frequently at this time. Taking good care of yourself is not self-indulgence; it's good sense. Often, the treatment for a fussy baby is more rest for the mother.

Recently, I came across a great idea that claims to help increase your breast milk supply in the form of "lactation cookies"—practical and delicious at the same time. You certainly don't need to spend a lot of money on them, but this recipe that you could bake comes from BellyBelly.com. au, written by Kelly Winder, and is one of their most popular articles (http://www.bellybelly.com.au/breastfeeding/breastmilk-supply-in-crease-breastmilk-lactation-cookie-recipe#.Ui8IlMZwqa8). I highly suggest you visit the page, as it includes lots of added information about women's experiences of eating them that might benefit you. Although they have reduced the recipe on their website in half, here is the original recipe:

Lactation Cookies

Ingredients:

- ► 2 cups self-raising whole wheat flour (if you have plain flour, add 1/2 tsp. baking powder)
- ► 1 cup butter or margarine
- ► 1 ½ cups brown sugar
- ► 4 tbsp. water
- ► 2 tbsp. flaxseed meal (or linseed, available in health food stores and some supermarkets)
- ► 2 large eggs
- ► 1 tsp. vanilla
- ► 1 tsp. baking soda
- ► 1 tsp. salt
- ► 3 cups oats, thick cut if available
- ► 1 cup or more chocolate chips/sultanas/almonds or anything else you like for added fun
- ► *2-4 tbsp. brewer's yeast – the secret ingredient, so don't substitute this

Preparation time: ~ 15 minutes

- ▸ Preheat oven to 350F / 180C
- ▸ Mix flaxseed meal and water, and set aside for 3 to 5 minutes. Cream, or beat well, the butter and sugar. Add eggs one at a time, and add with vanilla and mix well. Stir flaxseed mixture and add to the butter mix. Beat until blended. Sift together the dry ingredients, except the oats and chips. Add to butter mixture, and stir in oats, then chips. Scoop or drop on to a baking sheet, either greased or lined with parchment paper. It might be easier with a scoop since the dough is crumbly. Bake for 10 to 12 minutes, depending on the size of the cookies, and how soft you like the middle. Makes ~6 dozen cookies. Eat some and store the rest for later.

Positions for Breastfeeding

Recently, my knowledge was expanded when I read the book *An Introduction to Biological Nurturing: New Angles on Breastfeeding* (2010) by Suzanne Colson, which introduced me to the concept of laid-back breastfeeding. Before that, I used to say there are four common positions for nursing. The **cradle** (or classic sitting) **position** for nursing has the mother seated with the baby in her lap, or on one of the new nursing pillows that mothers wear that supports the baby's weight at just the right height while breastfeeding. When I was visiting my daughter after my grandson was born, we laughed that it reminded us of the old cigarette girls in nightclubs who carried their smoking materials around on such a platter. Before these became available, it was advised that a mother using the cradle position place the baby on top of a pillow in her lap so that she does not have to support all of the baby's weight on her arm.

A variation of the cradle position, and the one most recommended now for sitting, is the **cross-cradle position**. The baby is lying horizontally across the mother's body while the mother holds the breast from below in a U shape on the same side that the baby will feed. The other arm is holding the baby in the position described above for the asymmetrical latch.

Lying down and nursing is a wonderful way to breastfeed during the late night and early morning feedings and allows the mother to doze while she is feeding. Not only does the mother get more rest, but the baby also calms down more when nursing in a lying down position. However, the position is not limited to those times of the day because it also works well as a break in the day to take the baby to bed and have a breather.

The third position for breastfeeding is the (American) **football/rugby position**, which has the baby's face in front, but the rest of the body is along the side of her body towards her back. If a woman has twins, this is an effective way for her to breastfeed both at the same time. If a woman has had a cesarean delivery, this is an effective way to nurse without putting any pressure on her abdomen, which can be very painful right after the surgery. It looks unusual, but appearances don't matter if the position works for feeding.

The last position is a more recent discovery for me and was shown to me by my daughter's midwife after my grandson was born. I call this the **breast-crawl position** and I'll describe this more in the next section on laid-back positioning. It puts babies in a vertical position on the reclining mother's belly, very much like the position the baby is in when they crawl up to the breast right after birth. Babies in this position find and latch on to the breast naturally on their own. This was shown to us as a good way to feed the baby when there are sore nipples, but is not limited to that circumstance because it is being promoted more generally for mothers as well.

Babies will feed on each breast at a slightly different angle, and being flexible about how to angle the baby on each breast will make for smoother nursing experiences. That can mean changing your positioning between each side if that is how the baby nurses best. With the help of a sling, it is also possible for the mother to walk around while she is nursing, with at least one hand free to do other things if necessary, including talking on the phone or checking social media.

Laid-Back Positioning

What I'm calling the breast-crawl position is what Suzanne Colson calls **"laid-back maternal postures."** This is part of the Biological Nurturing (BN) she advocates as an evidence-based approach to breastfeeding. She says, "The BN maternal postures open the mother's body, increasing mother-baby behaviors, aiding latch and sustaining milk transfer" (Colson, 2010, preface). This kind of positioning ensures that mothers are at a comfortable angle, and the baby is face-down on top of them, with their weight on the mother's body and not on her arm(s), *another way of making the experience of nursing more comfortable.* The position activates both the mother's and baby's reflexes, and also frees up the mom's hands (without the sling mentioned above). This is how other mammals feed: on their tummies. The beauty of Colson's approach to breastfeeding is we don't have to teach mothers how to breastfeed, something that is truly changing the paradigm.

Colson's book is a way to demedicalize breastfeeding from all the (usually male) expert advice that has created interference with the process of nursing our babies. BN fosters maternal confidence as these postures release rewarding behaviors, and we tend to do things that we find enjoyable. As an activity of daily living, breastfeeding: "does not require professional help or routine management" (Colson, 2010, p. 20). Her book mentions the work done by Kittie Frantz, RN in California, who has been an expert advocate for breastfeeding for over 45 years. When I lived and worked as a childbirth educator in California, Kittie was attached to the birth center where a lot of my clients were giving birth. She produced a video of the breast crawl with a colleague who researched the effects of early mother/baby separation after birth in 1990, and it is one of the first such videos. One research finding was the maternal body provides continuity from fetus to neonate, what Colson calls a bridging strategy. Kittie's website slogan gets to the heart of the matter: *"Remember you are not managing an inconvenience, you are raising a human being."*

The two main components of Biological Nurturing are:

1. A range of maternal laidback sitting postures, where the pelvic support is sacral, and not "typist" sitting.

2. A range of baby positions, also called neonatal lie, in different directions: lying up and down, across, or obliquely on top of mom's body.

There is so much more useful information packed into this book, which has changed the thinking around breastfeeding, that I'm unable to include in this section. Although the book seems to be geared towards the

breast and completely emptying it first before you offer the second. Pump or express to comfort, but don't empty your breasts, or they will continue making more milk. Your supply will eventually adapt to your baby's needs. If all else fails, a couple of Altoids or some sage will lower your supply. But use with caution; you don't want to lower your supply completely.

Expressing milk can sometimes heal sore nipples unless the mom has a yeast infection (thrush) on her breasts that is causing soreness. The first thing to do with sore nipples is to address the possible causes: latch difficulties, anatomical issues in the baby's mouth (tongue-tie), or infection. Remedies for treating them will be based on what the issue is. Lanolin or hydrogel dressings provide relief (but don't address the cause), and some people like peppermint water too. People who have allergies to wool may react to lanolin.

I experienced soreness with both my second child and also with my last child. Although there was no engorgement with my fourth child, he did breastfeed in a way that seemed to maul the inside of my right breast. He had a strong suck, what I would laughingly call an institutional Hoover, and if I hadn't had experience with nursing, I could easily have given up with the pain that I felt while nursing. But I knew it would go away, and it did in a matter of weeks, and it gave me a better understanding of how easy it is to give up when things are challenging. Patience and perseverance are what help in times like this. However, you want to get skilled lactation care, and if the problem doesn't resolve, then see someone else. Pain indicates a problem as I'll discuss next. "This too shall pass" is a great motto for a new mother with sore nipples. In fact, it's a good motto for parenting in general.

Pain

There is a wide range of possible causes for nipple or breast pain during lactation, but if it's more than a twinge, find help as soon as possible because that indicates an issue that needs attention. Positioning and breast attachment are the main causes of nipple pain, and tongue-tie (ankyloglossia) is another cause, affecting about five percent of the population because the baby is unable to move the tongue to draw milk out properly when the frenulum is short or thick. It can also be caused by an infection, such as candida (yeast) or a staph infection. Viruses, such as herpes simplex and zoster, also cause pain. Another little miracle of nursing is how babies' saliva changes in response to an infection, activating maternal antibodies to it. When women are breastfeeding, and their baby develops thrush (yeast) inside their mouths with patchy white areas, it's highly probable that this will be transmitted to the mother, causing her pain. It didn't affect me when my daughter had it (and we gave her liquid lactobacillus culture as treatment), but it did affect her when her son was born.

Vasospasm in the nipple can cause sharp pain in the breast. This can be caused by damage to the nipples from a shallow latch or tongue-tie, or autoimmune conditions, such as lupus or rheumatoid arthritis. Some prescription medications can help with vasospasm, but the first thing to do is address any issues with the latch. A poor latch/suck dynamic can be painful when there is suboptimal positioning, leading to a shallow latch and abnormal compression of the nipple. Plugged ducts are another cause of pain. Because pain is a common cause of early breastfeeding cessation, it is a good idea to have an evaluation done by a lactation specialist to address the cause of the pain. Anything longer than one or two feeds is too long. There are lots of resources now to address this promptly.

There are a variety of medical treatments for pain, depending on its cause. You want to rule out tongue-tie, infection, latch issues, or an underlying medical condition. When there is a staph infection, seek medical treatment, or it can spiral into something serious. For the cases that don't require medical attention, I always prefer holistic and behavioral strategies, like warm compresses, massage therapy, not pumping or expressing milk if there's an overabundance, expressing milk if there are blocked ducts, and taking lactobacillus culture for yeast infections. There also seems to be a link between breast pain and mood disorders, because pain increases inflammation, which then increases the risk of depression, and this is true for all types of pain.

Finding a professional lactation consultant is easier these days than when I was having babies and when my clients needed help. Not all lactation consultants are created equal, and I've heard stories about women's experiences where the consultants, through their attitude and tactics, only made things worse; they left the mother feeling like a failure if the counseling didn't work. You want to look for an International Board Certified Lactation Consultant (IBCLC) who practices in your area. To become an IBCLC, there is a comprehensive training program that a practitioner must complete.

You want to find someone who is flexible, warm, compassionate, up to date in knowledge that is ever expanding, and considers your specific circumstances. There is no such thing as a one-size-fits-all approach to breastfeeding counseling. Maybe you can find someone that another mother recommends. If you are not getting good help, look for someone else who meets the needs you have and is a good fit for you. If the lactation consultant is part of an organization, think about reporting your negative experience so that other women don't end up having the same bad experience. You will help them improve their services, and maybe the training of lactation consultants.

La Leche League International is one way to go, offering free advice and group meetings that cover a wider variety of topics. In the UK, there are a variety of free breastfeeding support organizations, such as the Association of Breastfeeding Mothers (ABM), Breastfeeding Network (BfN), the NCT (National Childbirth Trust), and La Leche League. In the U.S., La Leche League, Women, Infants, and Children (WIC), and Breastfeeding USA are peer-support programs that empower women to nurse their babies. WIC is the largest source of support in the U.S. LLLI also have a helpline in the U.S.: **877-4LALECHE**. Peer support is also growing around the world to help breastfeeding mothers, and baby cafes are great for that. Get the help you need so that you can settle into a positive nursing experience.

CHAPTER 13

Advantages of Breastfeeding

Comparing Breast Milk and Cows'-Milk Formula

Before discussing the advantages of breastfeeding, it is useful to draw some comparisons between human milk and formula. I've developed the table below as a visual that compares and contrasts the different substances, and this table has evolved over the years as we continue to learn more about the elements of human milk. I've included the essentials, and you can find other sources that get even more elaborate in the breakdown of human milk and formula, including individual vitamins and minerals, such as, https://www.thehealthcloud.co.uk/formula-vs-breastfeeding/. I chose this website because it has a table of comparison, whereas others don't.

My explanations on the content of this table will follow below it.

Comparison of Breast Milk and Cow's-Milk formula

Components and Processes	Breast Milk	Cow's-Milk Formula
Protein	Lactalbumin – important for brain cells	Casein – important for muscles
	11g per liter	33g per liter
The coefficient of utilization (how the body assimilates it)	90%	75%
Iron	Lactoferrin	Synthetic iron – does not absorb when in milk

milk aids in calcium absorption, helping to utilize proteins easily and completely. The other sugars in cows' milk (galactose, glucose, and others in addition to lactose) cause the intestinal tract to be too alkaline. This is an ideal medium for the growth of harmful bacteria and organisms, which is what causes foul smelling stools.

Formula-fed babies excrete large quantities of unused calcium and phosphorous in their stool, and human milk has one-quarter of the amount of calcium in it, and it is completely absorbed. Babies fed cows'-milk formula grow larger and heavier skeletons than breastfed babies.

Colostrum, the first milk substance that is secreted by the breasts, protects against allergies and strengthens the immune system. Formula often causes allergies and taxes the immune system. There are important antibodies in breast milk, such as Lactobacillus Bifidus, to protect the intestines, and growth factors, peptides, and natural hormones in breast milk that don't exist in formulas. Natural vitamins are part of human milk, but the vitamins in formula are artificially injected. The fat content is different too. Skin-to-skin contact is built into giving human milk, offering the warmth of the body along with the milk. Many formula-feeding mothers also feed with skin-to-skin contact. The efficiency of human milk is a true advantage of breastfeeding in and of itself.

The Biological Norm of Breastfeeding

Physical Advantages for the Baby

The value of colostrum cannot be overstated, with its many protective and healing properties, and how it prepares the body to function. Colostrum has an oily, yellowish, thick texture to it and it resembles blood more than milk. It helps gut closure through the presence of the IgA (Immunoglobulin A) antibody, making the lining of the intestinal walls impermeable to large molecules, as the cell junctions seal up in the first few days. It affects the mucous membrane of the intestine, which is most permeable at this stage, sensitizing it to foreign proteins.

Cows'-milk formulas and pathogens have large molecules, and allergy occurs when whole-protein molecules, unfamiliar to the body's chemistry, are absorbed through the bowel in those first few days. This, potentially, throws the body into an autoimmune response. Antibodies are then produced to attack and digest this foreign material. Rapid gut closure, initiated by colostrum, protects against allergy and against attacking pathogens. Colostrum also contains disease antibodies, particularly for viral diseases, such as polio, and many *staphylococci*, and *E. coli*, in higher concentration than in blood serum. These antibodies are not transferred through the placenta.

Certain active white blood cells (lymphocytes and macrophages) in colostrum sweep the gastrointestinal tract clean of infectious microorganisms and foreign material. Colostrum has unusually high concentrations of vitamins A and E as protection against infection. Colostrum has a laxative effect and brings on the first meconium stools, further cleaning out the bowel, while eliminating all the meconium in the body. The frequent feeding of colostrum to a baby brings the mature milk in sooner, supplying the needed fluid to control levels of bilirubin, which can cause jaundice. Need-feeding (responding to the baby's needs) maintains bilirubin levels at a healthy range that is protective and not excessive.

Breast milk itself is also antibacterial, having its immune-enhancing qualities, while also providing the healthy bacteria that are a vital part of the microbiome. With a variety of autoimmune diseases on the rise in the 21st century, this is extremely important. Researchers from Duke University have discovered that breast milk antibodies help to neutralize HIV in infected mothers when they are exclusively nursing, inhibiting the transmission of the virus that causes AIDS to almost 0. The research was done because only 10% of HIV-infected nursing mothers pass the virus to their infants, and the research probed the immune response that protected 90% of babies (http://www.sciencedaily.com/releases/2012/05/120522152653. htm). When mothers mixed-feed, the baby has a much higher risk for contracting HIV, and therefore, the recommendation in industrialized countries may remain that HIV-infected mothers avoid breastfeeding. For those mothers who choose to breastfeed, the course of action is to also continue with combined antiretroviral therapy (cART) along with exclusive breastfeeding.

The *Lactobacillus Bifidus* factor in breast milk creates byproducts that strengthen the intestinal tract against the growth of microorganisms and maintains an acid environment, which is hostile to bacteria, but which promotes the growth of safe and protective intestinal flora. This is nature's probiotic. Human milk is a major source of GLA (gamma linolenic acid), the direct precursor to prostaglandins 1, one of the groups of cell regulators present in nearly all cells and body tissues.

To sum up the physical advantages for the baby, human milk is protective against allergies and infections in both the digestive and respiratory systems. It can be digested rapidly and easily, is raw and fresh at all times, diapers/nappies are less smelly since most of it is used and less excreted, and there are fewer skin disorders, and less eczema and diaper/nappy rash, which are often allergic reactions.

Physical Benefits for the Mother

There are physiological benefits to the mother as well. During birth, breast-feeding, or just having contact with the nipple, keeping it erect, will assist with the delivery of the placenta. Nursing lessens the chance of postpartum hemorrhage since with each nursing, the uterus contracts and becomes firm. This contracting of the uterus speeds the process of involution, bringing the uterus back to its non-pregnant size and shape. "After pains," which feel like heavy menstrual cramps, are a healthy sign from your body that involution is happening. You can make some homemade rice or lavender packs that you can put into the freezer or microwave that will help with afterpains. We covered (in Part 2) how, as long as you remain the sole source of nourishment for the baby (meaning no other food substances or pacifiers have been introduced), then nursing provides relative contraceptive protection. However, as soon as other foods or formula are introduced, or your baby starts sleeping through the night, pregnancy is possible. Some women do ovulate, even when exclusively nursing, so it is a good idea to use the extra protection of a barrier form of contraception.

Emotional and Maternal Benefits

The advantages are not just physical. Breastfeeding impacts on your emotional state too, and the emotional benefits are equally satisfying and important. A new mother's emotions are labile, another way of saying what I said in Part 1; your emotions are all over the place in the early postpartum period. This can include crying, poor concentration, and exhaustion. Nursing answers many deep-seated emotional needs that enable you to be more responsive to your baby.

Part of this comes from prolactin, which we described in Part 2 as being responsible for the production of milk and, together with oxytocin, triggers mothering behaviors in women. Breastfeeding fosters attachment, as each nursing period renews the hormonal cocktail that influences the desire to stay connected, strengthening the maternal/infant bond, while expressing affection through intimate, tactile contact. It brings you into a deeper experience of your femininity. The baby's emotional needs are met through immediate response to its hunger cries, with no delays to make bottles, and regular skin contact, which is the first language of communication. The skin is the most developed sensory organ at birth, and this contact will lead to a healthy sense of body awareness beginning at birth.

Seeds of intimacy

The vast majority of women born during the babyboom generation were *not* breastfed. This generation of women, including me, didn't have the personal cellular memory for this experience, which would have helped in choosing this for our children. I believe some of the social consequences of missing out on breastfeeding are manifest in a society that has become alienated and isolated in its inability to express love and intimacy, especially with the recent surge of hatred, bigotry, racism, and misogyny on full display in 2018.

The babyboom generation was also the one to re-embrace breastfeeding again, and I successfully breastfed four children, and the last two were breastfed for two years each. The seeds of intimacy are sown during skin-to-skin contact, the buzzwords that started with kangaroo care in the 1990s, and recently, in maternity wards advocating for this contact right after birth. This body contact is our introduction to physical closeness, which develops into a strong ability to have close relationships later in life. This language of the skin translates into increased abilities to communicate with others, personally and intimately.

I have always believed that if all women breastfed and relaxed into this experience of nurturing, our children as a generation could then reverse the trends that we see all too often in the headlines. I know it cannot solve all the problems in society, but it is a step in the right direction. I discuss this in Part 4.

Our Capacity to be Intimate and Connected

Once the seeds of intimacy are sown, it is important to tend to these fragile seedlings as they grow into a stronger connectedness with others. Intimacy is a growing edge for most people, and with an inhibited experience of it growing up, many people aren't comfortable being intimate with others. It is hard to share the deepest parts of ourselves, and it can feel much easier just to stay inside and not reach out. All the stimulation that is purchased through toys and equipment, along with programs for babies, cannot substitute for the essential tactile stimulation that babies need. The rest is compensation.

In the next Part on Bonding and Attachment, I discuss attachment parenting, which evolved out of attachment theory into a style of parenting. You don't have to buy into the whole attachment-parenting experience to be physically close to your baby. I believe too many mothers today are approaching the process of mothering with a black-or-white attitude. It is not an either/or experience; it's both/and. You need to feel free to pick and choose the bits that resonate with you.

Nurturing the mother allows partners to access some of their feminine qualities within, as all of us are a composite of both masculine and feminine characteristics. The nursing couple is a mutually beneficial relationship in which both the mother and baby benefit on physical, emotional, and relational levels, and this interdependence is undeniable. The past emphasis on oversized masculinity in men, which inhibited the expression of sensitivity, has changed with each new generation of men. Although some fathers feel excluded by breastfeeding, they could instead appreciate the opportunity that nursing gives the mother to be more receptive, both as a mother and a lover. This makes the circle of unity more complete.

Breastfeeding as a Sexual Expression

In a woman's life, the hormone oxytocin flows throughout her bloodstream during orgasm, pregnancy, birth, and breastfeeding, and now we know this goes beyond these special circumstances too. All of these experiences comprise a woman's full expression of sexuality, although birth seems to have been stripped of that dimension when it was brought into hospitals. As a birth professional, I have found that often, someone who is inhibited in her erotic activities is also likely to be inhibited during birth, and modest and inhibited about nursing.

The way in which obstetrics is practiced makes it difficult to experience birth as a sexual happening. If a laboring woman is encouraged to make noise during her labor, it often sounds the same as the sounds made during lovemaking. In both circumstances, there is a great release of tension, so if she is a noisy lovemaking person, chances are that it would be appropriate for her to make noise while giving birth too.

Oxytocin has a natural relaxing effect on the body, like the feeling after an orgasm that allows a couple to fall asleep in each other's arms. During lactation, oxytocin is what helps us get through the stress of newborn parenting and its constant demands on energy. It can be an island of serenity every couple of hours. Wouldn't it be a real reversal to see each feeding as an opportunity to chill out, rather than an imposition on personal time? Here we have a perfect example of going with the flow.

Although nursing is not viewed as being connected to our sexual identity, biochemically, the experience is the same. When breastfeeding, the suction created by the baby's mouth, once latched, is quite different than breast play during lovemaking, but some women find that they experience great sensual pleasure during nursing. The sensuality is built into it by the skin contact alone, and the tendency to be stroked and touched by the baby as it feeds is also a mutually sensuous activity. Through breastfeeding, our babies get the message of life-affirming love, and that bodies are for enjoyment, not destruction. Breastfed babies learn healthy pleasure, trust, and love in the arms of their mothers.

Breastfeeding brings us into heart-to-heart contact with another. People learn different ways of communicating love: love for our mate, love for our children, and the two are distinct forms of expression, but of equal intensity. When we expand the definition of sexuality to include more than just our erotic experiences, we understand it to be the full expression of ourselves as creative beings. It is a vibration that moves us to join not only bodies, but hearts, minds, and spirits as well. Orgasmic birth recognizes that birth can be sexual. Nursing serves this purpose too, and lactation is a very creative endeavor. Not only is this a sensual experience for you, but it is sensory stimulation for the baby as well and the continuation of the closeness, which was a biological unit until birth.

A pattern of love and sensuality is being imprinted on the consciousness of the baby when at the breast, and loving, non-seductive caressing of children is the ultimate sex education. A structure for mutuality is created, laying the foundation for strong self-esteem. When babies develop a healthy sense of trust, it translates into an increased ability to relate to others intimately. Babies become whole human beings able to trust the moment and surrender into it.

The Emotional After Effects of Weaning[1]

While writing this book, I learned that many women experience some emotional anguish once they wean their babies from breastfeeding. I was aware that it affected me after my last two children finished nursing (my first child was nursed for 7 months, and my second child breastfed for 5 months). Although my last two children were 2 years old when they weaned, and the process was done over a long period, I felt the loss of intimacy that nursing my children offered. I did not ascribe my feelings to hormonal changes because the gradual weaning process over many months meant steadily diminishing levels of oxytocin and prolactin, not a sudden drop off. I was ready to have my body back and to be free from the constant consideration of my child that breastfeeding required. And I felt sad about the loss of closeness and connection that breastfeeding provided. I also had a sense that I needed to affirm my femininity once again in other ways.

Their newfound independence was a joy and a sorrow. Like so many other complex feelings after having a baby, the mixed emotions surprised me, realizing that the experience of breastfeeding was now in the past. I felt that way after my daughter, my third child, weaned. We had been more or less connected at the hip (as well as the breast!) during those years as a nursing couple. I felt a little wistful during the last feeding, thinking this was my last

---

1   For those where weaning has a double meaning of stopping breastfeeding (U.S.) or introducing solids (UK), my use of the word here is the American version for breastfeeding cessation.

child and I'd never do this again. Then years later, we were inspired to have a fourth child, and I was glad for another chance to have that closeness. When he weaned, I knew this was definitely the last time, and I suffered the loss. I felt I had a solid bond with my children through the nursing experience, but the cuddly feeling of having my child (no longer a baby) in body contact was finished. The physical oneness was over. The freedom to drink alcohol and the relief of restored physical independence was countered by the nostalgia for a special close relationship between mother and infant/child.

The benefits of breastfeeding that are discussed in depth in this Part, like relaxation and calm, are no longer available and some mothers will feel more agitated and anxious when they have weaned. The anti-inflammatory effects of the hormones are now lost, and levels of stress can increase. Though the emotions of weaning don't get much attention in the public sphere, weaning can be associated with depression, called post-weaning depression. It doesn't usually have the same impact or last as long as postpartum depression, but it is a real phenomenon that mothers notice. Generally, it resolves on its own. However, we need to be aware that weaning has emotional side effects and be prepared for those by finding support from our partner and friends, giving valuable attention to our babies in other ways that replace the nursing experience, and reaching out to others. No need to suffer in silence. When I used to attend La Leche League meetings in California and New York, the weaning session was the most popular, and mothers would attend with children of all ages. I don't remember the subject of emotional responses to weaning brought up at those weaning meetings I attended.

Early weaning is a different story from the one that I've told because there are likely to be greater hormonal shifts to navigate in the beginning months. It can feel traumatic for mother and baby when it's done too abruptly. Then there's the possibility that the baby is not ready to wean, and cries for mother's milk relentlessly. And mother might not be ready when the child self-weans. There's such a range of experiences with weaning. The most notable issue is when mothers are unable to continue nursing, and there is a wide range of problems that can cause this. Some feel a terrible loss and a certain level of incompetence at what they perceive to be their failure to feed their babies, and others are relieved to be able to switch to formula feeding and move on. They may not notice the after effects of weaning because there are so many other emotions playing into the mix.

I spoke to "Emma" who had two children who had weaned: the first at 1 year and the second at 6 months. She felt that something changed with the weaning process, and talked about how the emotional regulation she had enjoyed changed with each dropped feeding. She experienced a period of depressed mood, missing the "physical sensation of not having hormones pumping to make you happy." The calmness she felt strongly when nursing was also missed as she weaned over a three to four months period. She was very sensitive to the sensations of oxytocin in her system, and equally so when it was gone. By the time her daughter was 10 months, she was only nursing two feeds a day, which dropped to one by 11 months. The baby's appetite for solids was so good that she was not so keen on nursing anymore. Even with a withdrawal over time, she felt the grief of ending the breastfeeding experience. She acknowledged feeling more energy within herself and noticed that she had more color in her cheeks after ending. However, she was pregnant again when her daughter turned one!

The second time around was a more complicated process overall. An early case of mastitis at 2 weeks meant the baby had to nurse on one side (the one he didn't like as much), causing an oversupply in one breast and an undersupply in the other breast. He was unhappy that his favorite side was out of action! After that resolved, later on, he would pull away from the breast, and after the breastfeeding period, he was diagnosed with type 1 diabetes, followed several months later with celiac disease, and Emma felt retrospectively that he was probably lactose intolerant earlier on. Once food was introduced, he was less interested in nursing, and Emma started weaning him when he was 4 months old. The loss of the "bubble of oxytocin" was depressing, and again she described the emotional regulation that breastfeeding provided, even with a more sudden weaning process. She too felt the sadness of stopping with her last child. Emma and I agree that oxytocin benefits the whole family, with its flavor of contentment and satisfaction. It's also a demonstration of the affiliative power of oxytocin when it's released into the air in a group of people who love each other. She said they all missed it a little bit when it was over.

When I asked Emma what advice she would give to new parents, she said, "Be aware that your body is producing something that sustains the element of contentment in you. You may feel a sense of loss or withdrawal, but know it's just an adjustment period and not something you have to be concerned with." She specified that for her that adjustment period lasted about two to three months. Whatever your experience of weaning is (and we've been concentrating more on the mother than the child), making quality time focused on your child's needs keeps those cuddles happening and keeps the bond between you strong. Some mothers advocate for exercise, a way of using that extra energy that Emma was talking about. I know the women who showed up at my postpartum exercise classes for 20 years enjoyed the blend of getting back into shape while feeling a community with other women in the same stage of life and supporting each other through the breastfeeding journey. If you can find that kind of postpartum gathering or program in your area, go for it. You'll be less likely to dwell on the sadness and more likely to look forward to the next stages of development for yourself and your child. Whether or not you find a group or class, go easy on yourself. This too shall pass.

CHAPTER 14

Cultural Perspectives Around Breastfeeding

In the 21st century, with the internet and social media, women can access information in a way that earlier generations couldn't. For a long time, women have been influenced by cultural perspectives around breastfeeding, but it has certainly intensified with the advent of social media. This chapter will discuss the cultural construction of the breastfeeding experience, and how many factors can impede this experience.

Professional Indifference

One contributing factor to the challenges of nursing is health care providers' limited understanding of this complex physiological process. As Grandma disappeared with the loss of extended families in the 20th century, the void was filled by the doctor/book combination of information and authority placed in experts. When a woman had concerns, the answers were given as medical prescriptions for social and emotional issues. I can still remember my pediatrician visiting me in the hospital and giving me a prescription note saying "feed every four hours."

Breastfeeding involves the whole body and mind, and is more than just a method of feeding. A mechanistic ideology comes from the idea that breasts (and for that matter, uteri) are like machines you can turn on and off. A certain rationalized indifference developed, as neither maternal nor infant-care professionals took responsibility for informing the mother. It's not something they learn about in medical school or specialized training, and the burgeoning medical literature on breastfeeding is something that is relatively recent. Breastfeeding, which is not an illness, is rarely featured in the medical curriculum. In fact, in the past, medical texts on reproduction have been known to have omitted any mention of breasts or breastfeeding.

Often, the major blocks to breastfeeding originate in the places we turn to for resources, the "experts" we encounter in hospitals, and our doctors (GPs and pediatricians). Because breastfeeding is not a subject studied in medical school or residency programs, and female pediatricians or GPs who have not breastfed can be negative role models for women who make certain assumptions based on the doctor's rejection of this process, you may experience a biased attitude from this person. However, it must be said that some doctors may have tried and couldn't do it. If a male doctor has a partner who has successfully breastfed, then there may be some limited personal experience. The illusion that pediatricians will have the answers on breastfeeding may not be true. However, in some places, you might find a pediatrician who is also a lactation consultant, and they have their professional organization, the Academy of Breastfeeding Medicine. Now that's an expert to prize!

Pediatricians once considered nursing to be part of women's reproduction, and therefore, part of the obstetric domain. This has been changing as the American Academy of Pediatrics has become a leader on breastfeeding policy, acknowledging this as part of their purview. Obstetricians related breastfeeding to the baby's hunger, and therefore, a pediatric concern, and this has also been evolving. Some OBs view this decision as being very personal and don't want to pressure women, as if vaginal birth is less personal. Whenever a problem would arise, the medical solution has traditionally been a bottle. A doula, lactation consultant, or peer counselor can offset this excessive reliance on doctors for knowledge they don't have.

The Breastfeeding Landscape

Once upon a time, the sight of a mother nursing her baby was a commonplace occurrence and people took it in their stride (this is true for some countries more than for others, as not all countries were breastfeeding friendly). Because it was a natural event and part of life, girls grew up expecting that they would feed their babies in the same way and would be surrounded by female role models who would provide the support they needed. More men had a balanced view of breasts as being functional for feeding babies in addition to being sexual objects.

The 20th century saw the removal of breastfeeding mothers from the landscape in many places (but thankfully, not all), relegated to the private sphere to be properly covered up, probably with the advent of bottle-feeding. There has been an experimental video floating around on Facebook recently comparing the reactions to a woman sitting on a bench with revealing cleavage, and another woman nursing her baby. The hostile response from people walking by to the nursing mother was shocking to witness. I'm a real advocate for nursing wherever it's necessary. It is a sad reality that some women who want to nurse their babies discreetly in public can be exposed to such hostile reactions from people unable to appreciate the value of nourishing our babies the way humans were designed to do it. These days, with the advent of social media, there is often a negative backlash when this kind of harassment goes public, something else you can see on Facebook posts.

I believe humanity needs to embrace the intimacy and love that is shared when a baby nurses at the breast, and spread an appreciation for that kind of connection as the antidote to war and aggression. The reversal of cultural hostility towards breastfeeding will only happen when we once again accept the sight of nursing mothers and babies doing what comes naturally, uninhibited by others and protected by laws that prohibit people from harassing mothers who breastfeed. The good news is there is legislation to protect mothers from this kind of provocation (as a civil-rights issue) in all 50 states. Also, social media will push back against situations that compromise mother's rights these days.

Our culture insists that "Breast is best, but we don't want to see it." Here's a loathsome quote from someone opposed to breastfeeding in public: "breastfeeding might be natural, but so is urinating and I don't do that in public." Those offended by the sight of functioning breasts are equating breast milk full of nutrients to waste products that are disposed of in separate areas for health and safety reasons (Brown, 2016). These mixed messages add to the confusion about infant feeding because breastfeeding breasts are not for public consumption, while deep décolletage is prized. Functioning breasts? Oh, no! Sexual breasts? Oh, yes! Facebook has some interesting rules about images of breastfeeding that I will discuss next, and those seem to reflect this view of what's "acceptable."

Cultural vs. Biological Femininity

I believe that one of the difficulties that women experience during breast-feeding is the pull between cultural femininity and biological femininity. This was first brought to my attention in Karen Pryor's book, *Nursing Your Baby* (1977). Cultural femininity is comprised of many stereotypes that limit a woman's expression of self, mold her personality, and affect her body image. Biological femininity is the expression of feminine power through our reproductive capacity which includes childbirth and breastfeeding.

When society began to glorify breasts for their sexual attractiveness rather than their function, the exposure of breasts became limited to private moments. We only show breasts to our partners, and not to anyone else. Such a taboo is bound to have an impact on the choice to breastfeed, and can also manifest as a stumbling block for those who do breastfeed. Why is it more acceptable to see nubile young women, glamorously dressed in décolletage that meets the waistline, but it's obscene to see a mother feeding her baby at the breast? This is a debate that is currently happening on Facebook, which routinely removes images of mothers' breastfeeding, but shows all manner of other sexualized images of breasts.

There is a cultural distortion in elevating the useless shape of the body curve as having more significance than the functional aspect of the glands. These glands have produced the perfect food to nourish our babies, like no other substance on earth. Society falls short of encouraging mothers to go the natural route in a practical way. Mothers who are unable to breastfeed experience huge disappointment and guilt at not being able to fulfill that potential, often because of ineffective encouragement and/or support to succeed. Lactation is the natural state of the mammary glands. Choosing not to breastfeed is the denial of this natural aspect of our maternity.

I am uniquely qualified to discuss this topic, having once been a Playboy bunny (talk about glorified sex objects!) and a nursing mother and it wasn't the size of my breasts in those days that got me the job! In fact, it was breastfeeding that increased their size, but there were ways of uplifting breasts in the costume to work in the Playboy Club. The recent death of Hugh Hefner reminded me of this paradox of femininity. I have personally experienced both cultural and biological femininity, there is no comparison. Biological femininity is defined by nature. Cultural femininity is defined by others. My feminism helped me to transcend the stereotypes of cultural femininity. Susan Brownmiller wrote the book, *Femininity* (1984), and with regard to breasts she sums it up perfectly: "...the cultural belief that breasts are primarily decorative and intrinsically provocative seems related historically in Western civilization to the elimination of the routine sight of breasts as a means of nourishing the young" (p. 44, emphasis added). I think it's time to see nursing paraphernalia, like nursing pads, pumps, or bras, in other media beyond parenting and baby magazines. We would be fostering an acceptance of our biological femininity to offset the limitations of cultural femininity. We would be expanding the consciousness of society to accept breastfeeding as the natural biological experience that it is and desexualize it. In that context, I believe women wouldn't manifest such difficulties when they choose to nurse their babies.

Facebook Purity and Prurience

In September 2015, I gave a presentation at a conference organized by Birthlight, a UK association dedicated to helping new families move through the perinatal period, using yoga as the ground on which healing and growth are actualized. My paper was called "Postnatal Bodies, Distorted Representations, and Mother's Real-Life Experiences." I discussed how the media has such a profound influence on how we perceive our bodies and selves in relation to the photoshopped images of celebrities who get back into shape within weeks. It is an impossible standard to achieve without personal trainers, private chefs, and other facilitators, and yet, new mothers feel the pressure to conform.

As part of the preparation for my speech, I began to research how Facebook was creating its form of censorship regarding breastfeeding images posted on the site, which it deemed were pornographic. After years of removing these posts as obscene, they received some pushback from mothers and Facebook group pages and communities were created, such as "Facebook vs. Breastfeeding," and "Hey Facebook, breastfeeding is not obscene!" Mothers have been banned from Facebook as punishment for posting pictures of themselves nursing their babies. These two groups have 10,000 and 13,000 members respectively, calling for Facebook to stop removing images, bullying breastfeeders, and classifying the images as obscene.

The social-media construction of mothers' bodies seems to devalue this natural expression of nourishment. I don't know that this has changed since Mark Zuckerberg became a father (married to a pediatrician). Over the last 10 years, this protest movement has been covered by the media, who quote Facebook spokesmen on the policy to remove images, but the impetus to do this comes from its prudish users: "The photos we act upon are almost exclusively brought to our attention by other users who complain."

An article from *The Guardian* in February 2012, written by Rowan Davies, sums up Facebook's attitude and the impact this policy has on mothers, and it is worth quoting here:

> The wearying insistence on the obscenity of ordinary lactation contributes strongly to a real-world culture in which breastfeeding, despite a thousand officially sanctioned leaflets and posters, is holed below the waterline. Healthcare professionals tell mothers that they simply must breastfeed; yet the public seems to add, "but we must never be aware of it." A society that is not prepared to accept the odd flash of nipple is a society that is not prepared to accept breastfeeding.
>
> And it matters what Facebook does about this … *Facebook is one of the most influential cultural mediators in the world.* In reflecting and promoting the belief that milky nipples are injurious to public morality, it gives succour to every shopping centre security guard who's ever told a nursing mother to put it away or leave the premises. A mother who is told by Facebook that her breastfeeding photos have been removed because her nipples were showing is quite likely to be humiliated, upset, and one step closer to giving up on breastfeeding (emphasis added) (Davies, 2012).

However, in March of 2015, Facebook claimed to have changed its rules about breastfeeding images with its new policy on nudity. The social network had updated a number of guidelines in its community standards about the content that it allows or bans. "We also restrict some images of female breasts if they include the nipple, but we always allow photos of women actively engaged in breastfeeding or showing breasts with post-mastectomy scarring."

https://www.facebook.com/communitystandards/objectionable_content
Normalizing the sight of breastfeeding is an important step in increasing the incidence of mothers who choose to breastfeed. Facebook is now replete with breastfeeding images posted by mothers, and as younger women and girls are exposed to the sight of nursing mothers, it becomes part of their normal experience. Nevertheless, I don't think that Facebook will be the trendsetter for that because they are still removing images and banning people for posting photos of breastfeeding, despite their new rules on nudity.

Wouldn't it be nice if the next generation of women, who were "groomed" by social media, had access to real breastfeeding representations in a way that could be internalized as a physical expectation within their body images? If that *did* come to pass, I could imagine that that generation would have more ease of breastfeeding, and fewer difficulties and complications.

Cultural Interferences

Recently, it seems that women's reproductive rights have been under attack by backward-looking white men (mostly) harkening back to a time (Ozzie and Harriet in the 1950s) when a woman's role remained subordinate to her partner's. Her attractiveness is overemphasized, and the functional aspects of motherhood are seen as unpleasant. Some societies are more considerate of the transition to parenthood and provide paid leave and other family-support measures that express the social value for this tender time in life. Most women do not realize that breast tissue that has functioned retains its shape much *longer* than breast tissue that hasn't. It is pregnancy that changes the breasts, not breastfeeding. Our cultural ignorance of breastfeeding before pregnancy is startling. This is a subject that should be an inherent part of any sexual and reproductive-health course in secondary school.

Another issue that I hear from mothers is the level of inconsistent and often contradictory information they receive from midwives and nurses in the hospital, and at home after. It's a good idea to ask the person advising if she has breastfed herself, although that doesn't guarantee anything. You can get excellent advice from someone who hasn't, and terrible advice from someone who has, but cannot support well. However, her ability to empathize can be crucial in resolving any initial ineptness you might feel. Often, when mothers are awkwardly attempting this function, they are given wrong information and inadequate support. Mother and baby suffer, and things go downhill from a poor beginning.

Lactation consultants are the professionals to consult when there are issues. Other helpful resources include peer support through La Leche League or WIC, and baby cafes can be a great place to get help and find a support network. This moves us away from expert advice to lived experience as an important source of support, especially for those who cannot afford expensive consultants.

Supplemental bottles of water or formula can disturb the rhythm of breastfeeding, though women are usually not in the hospital long enough these days to experience this interference. I find it astounding that women have mammary glands that activate, begin production of milk forms, and flow into the breasts within days of the baby's birth. Nature's design is an exquisite plan. We do not produce milk without the means to express it. Trust that you will be able to figure it out. Surround yourself with those who can allay your doubts and fears, and support your efforts, such as partners/fathers, and friends who have succeeded in nursing.

A Summary of Breastfeeding

Prolactin and oxytocin are the primary hormones produced for breastfeeding. Their side effects cause a definitive mothering inclination. This means we are more responsive to our babies when prolactin causes the restless, anxious effects it does. It makes it almost impossible to ignore a crying baby. Then, when the baby latches on and the milk comes in (with oxytocin coming from the pituitary gland), the oxytocin causes the restorative effect of naturally tranquilizing us. The bottle-feeding mother does not benefit from this calming influence, but if she practices skin to skin, the skin releases oxytocin from the brain stem, which is more powerful than the milk-ejection reflex.

CHAPTER 15

Supporting Breastfeeding

*For Fathers/Partners/ Grandmothers to Read

Father/Partner Support for Breastfeeding

Breastfeeding is a team effort. If as fathers/partners, you are having any resistance to your partner's breastfeeding, see if you can find the courage to open the subject up for communication before she gives birth. If a mother suspects your disapproval, she will manifest different reasons why it doesn't work. If she feels that you are withholding your support or love for her, this can manifest as complications that can end in terminating the process. If the vibes she is picking up tell her you are hesitant or uncertain, unconsciously, the message will activate energy to increase *your* comfort. If she perceives that her choice to breastfeed is uncomfortable to you as the father/partner, or she is very stressed, then she can fix that by inhibiting her let-down reflex (unconsciously), or mastitis (breast inflammation), reduction in milk supply, sore nipples, or other ways to fail.

None of this happens at the conscious level, but if she senses that breastfeeding is a problem for you, she'll find ways to abandon it. As an intimate experience of life, it needs to be shared. Mothers need your *expressed* support to get over the initial hurdles that will come up in the beginning. I advise that partners take an active role in helping her out—to be there for her. If she senses your strong support for her choice and knows you are there for her when times are difficult, then she can begin to rally confidence around her maternal instincts.

It's a challenge for women to succeed at breastfeeding when they perceive disapproval or distaste for the idea from their partners. If the choice to breastfeed is going to compromise the other areas of your sexuality, is it worth it? Without cultural support, it is hard to persist. We end up trading one sexual facet of our nature for another. Sometimes, the only way that a woman can have a rewarding experience of nursing her baby is with active, vocal support from her partner. Any ambivalence, lack of enthusiasm, or indifference can have the effect of thwarting efforts to breastfeed. Most partners have no idea how crucial their input is to the success of nursing. She has to know that it's entirely all right and in order with you.

Fathers/partners are an important foundation for effective breastfeeding. Your guidance and strength are the cornerstones of happy feeding. Mothers also need your protection against the unintentional undermining of the nursing experience by people who are ignorant, asking questions like "are you sure you have enough milk?" or making a comment like, "maybe the baby's not getting enough." It's a form of verbal harassment, though it is usually *without* any malice. When she hears you declare her right to be a nursing mother and shielding her from such questions and comments, she can relax her defenses and mellow into happy nursing.

Recently, I came across another book that opened my eyes to the benefits of grandmother support too, and it's called *The Importance of Dads and Grandmas to the Breastfeeding Mother* (2017), written by Wendy Jones. It's chock-full of information that can enlighten grandmothers and partners about how breastfeeding works and how they can be the best support to their children and grandchildren, rather than making comments as I've just mentioned above that undermine the mother. The book is geared to the loved ones who surround the new mother, and it's full of tips, take-home messages, and suggestions of things to do to help. It even has a chapter on how to bottle-feed. An informed partner or grandparent is a true gift to the nursing mother. The book is wholly aligned with my view that expressed emotional and practical support is essential to happy and successful breastfeeding.

Confidence is a primary attribute for the success of breastfeeding. Our belief that we can do it is what makes it happen. Whenever a woman tells me that she's going to *try* to do it, I know it's likely that she'll fail.

After all, trying is effort without accomplishment. She lacks faith in her ability to succeed; she's tentative and unsure. Her emotional insecurity can play into feeding difficulties. We need to turn around our limiting beliefs about breastfeeding so that we can appreciate the incredible potential that nursing provides: the development of intimacy, the healthy benefits of human milk for the baby, the achievement of nourishing our babies, and the fulfillment of the postpartum experience in which breasts are filled with milk. Otherwise, the result can be what Niles Newton (1963) in her classic book, *Maternal Emotions*, called "unsuccessful breastfeeding." Although this quote is more than 50 years old, unfortunately, it also describes the contemporary experience for many modern mothers.

> Unsuccessful breastfeeding is a type of breastfeeding that is typical of the modern urban American mother. This type of breastfeeding is a difficult and tenuous process. There is constant worry about whether there is enough milk for the baby. The mother is expected to regulate her diet, her sleep, and her habits of living to help make her milk good and plentiful. She worries about washing her nipples, and about which breast to give, and when and how long to give it …Often the supply of milk is so insufficient that bottles must be resorted to supplement the breast milk. Breast abscesses and engorgement, and nipple fissures and erosions frequently cause extreme pain. The pain, the work, and the worry of unsuccessful breastfeeding make early weaning part of the unsuccessful breastfeeding pattern (Newton, 1963, p. 49).

This is something to avoid. By simplifying your life and preparing for the challenges of nursing, you can have the positive experience that you want.

Heart to Heart

The Neurovascular Reflex Points are situated around the head, neck, and throat, and boost circulation of both the blood and energy for the whole body and the brain. They can be used to eliminate the emotional and mental effects of stress. There is a point at the top of the head that is called the Heart Neurovascular Reflex Point, which we are going to pair with the heart chakra to help you feel grounded and calm, and to balance your hormones. Place one hand palm down and your other hand on top of it, also palm down, and then interlace your thumbs and your little fingers so that there are three fingers above and three fingers below.

First, place your hands at the top of your head in the center and hold them there for three to five minutes. Then, take your hands and place them over the heart, and hold them there for three to five minutes, elbows tucked in at your sides. In this way, you are moving the energies from your head to your heart because breastfeeding is a heart-centered experience, not a head trip. You can do it sitting, standing, or lying down. Not only does it calm the mind, but it's also good if there are problems in the feet.

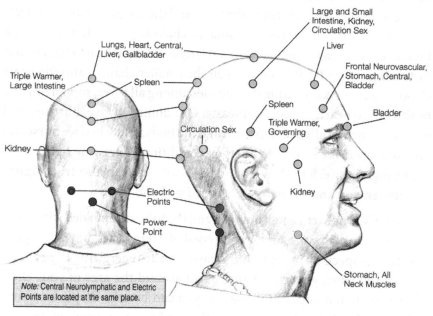

**Neurovascular Holding Points © 2009
Innersource, Inc., used by permission.**

Nine Hearts Exercise

This is one of my favorite energy medicine techniques, and it helps to open your Radiant Circuits, which we will talk more about in the next part on Bonding and Attachment. This gets all the radiant circuits flowing and has an impact on the heart. We start off doing three hearts around the face, then three hearts around the torso, and then three hearts around your entire body. Always exhale through the mouth any time you are doing energy movements. Starting with your hands on the front of your thighs for grounding, take a deep breath in and out. While inhaling, move your hands up the center of your body to the top of the forehead. Exhaling, trace a heart from your forehead to your chin. Move your fingers up the center of your face, leading with the middle finger while inhaling.

When exhaling, trace another heart, and repeat the sequence a third time.

Breathing deeply, slowly move your hands to the middle of your chest over the heart chakra. Inhaling, trace a heart with flattened hands moving up over the chest and while exhaling, tracing the heart around the breasts, down the trunk and inside the hips bones, and ending at the top of the pubic bone. Repeat this two more times, starting from the pubic bone and tracing up to the chest while inhaling, and tracing down around the torso on the exhale.

The largest hearts are traced from the top of the pubic bone, drawing flat hands up the body to the heart chakra as you inhale. Exhaling, turn your hands so that the fingertips touch and the palms lie on the top of the chest. Inhaling, bring the hands into a prayer position and raise them above your head. Separate your hands while lifting them higher, and turn the palms out and place the backs of hands together.

While exhaling very slowly and forcefully, slowly press the outstretched arms down to your sides as if you are pushing down weight, and continue to bring the hands down the sides of the legs or all the way down to your feet. Draw two more giant hearts this way. Feel free to improvise by tracing hearts wherever you want, including on your baby.

Spleen Tap

Spleen meridian helps with milk production, and for this chapter, we will work with Spleen as a radiant circuit, sometimes called the "mother of upbeat mom energy" (Eden & Feinstein, 2012b). There are four meridians that are also radiant circuits, and Spleen is one of them. You want to keep things flowing in Spleen, which will then maintain the flow of milk production on an energetic level too.

The Spleen Tap is done by creating a three-finger notch with the thumb, index, and middle fingers, and tapping on the point that is one rib below the bra, in line with the nipples. You will often feel a little tenderness there, and this is true for all people since Spleen is often depleted by Triple Warmer (we talked about this in the last part). Tap both sides simultaneously for 15 to 30 seconds.

Tracing Spleen Meridian

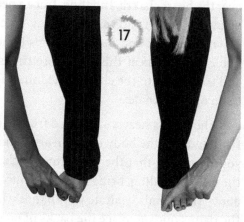

By tracing the path of the Spleen meridian, you can activate it as a radiant circuit. Starting at the lower corner of the big toenail (on the bunion side), **#17,** use your hands to trace up the inside of the legs to the groin, flaring out with your hands to your hips, and moving up the sides of the body to the armpit, and then down again to the bottom of your rib cage. This end-point is called **Spleen 21** (this location is shown in Part 1). This simple action gets the flow going through Spleen and, therefore, the flow going for milk production too.

Connecting Heaven and Earth

This was covered in the Daily Energy Routine in Chapter 5, and again, in the last part on hormones. However, it activates Spleen as a radiant circuit, so keep doing it. See the instructions in Chapter 1.

To Sum Up

Between the heart and spleen, you will be bathed in loving energy and assisted with processing energies of thought, experience, and emotion, as well as food, so that you can enjoy a state of harmony and balance. The period of breastfeeding is a short one in the greater span of one's life. I spent five years of my life nursing my four children. It helps to be in the mother mode when the baby's born. Don't rush to be somewhere else. The number of times you'll know this experience in life is limited.

In the 21st century, there has been a tidal shift in consciousness towards love, and breastfeeding is a great training ground for a mother and baby. Our heart opens up when we embrace our child at the breast. Mothers commonly feel more comfortable nursing on the left side, where the heart chakra is more developed. Nursing babies are known to become more confident in their bodies as a result of this early experience of physical contact. These children grow up with a healthy, accepting attitude toward bodies based on the language of the skin to which they were initiated. A social byproduct would be a reduction in self-consciousness, allowing more girls who come of age to approach breastfeeding with confidence and trust. If the first experience in life is to have been embraced at the breast, many mothers will carry that memory with them into their desire to continue this legacy.

A beautiful quote comes from Sam Keen, from his powerful book, *The Passionate Life* (1983):

> In the natural course of things, the rupture caused by birth is healed immediately. Mother takes the child, still connected to her through the oxygen-rich umbilical cord, to her breast. In her arms, a complex bond is woven from the touch of skin, the smell of breath, the sound of voice, the benediction of smiles, the rhythm of rocking, the resonance of the beating heart, the taste of the breast. There is immediate hormonal and sensory knowledge. This is *my* mother. The key fits the lock. Our first cognition is recognition (p. 40).

Breastfeeding is a wonderful experience of connection with another human being and sows the seeds of intimacy at the start of life so that children learn how to connect positively with others throughout life. May you be blessed with a happy and contented breastfeeding experience.

In the next Part, I will explore the experiences of bonding and attachment, practices that have been getting a lot of attention from the media, and from parents themselves.

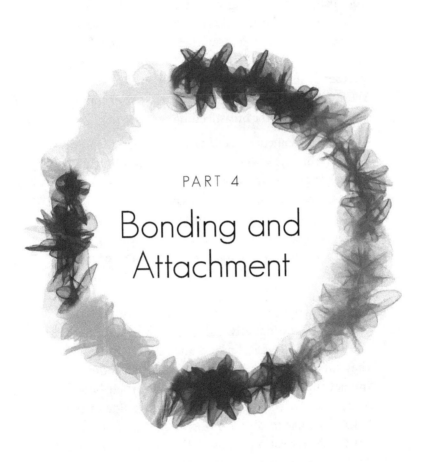

PART 4

Bonding and
Attachment

PART 4 INTRODUCTION

In Part 4, we explore what bonding and attachment are so you can understand what is involved, and maximize the experiences that will enhance your connection with your baby. Both bonding and attachment are processes that unfold with time, allowing you and your baby to connect in an intimate way that lays the foundation for your child's future significant relationships. Your partner is also bonding and attaching to the baby in these early months, in various ways that encourage intimacy beyond the breastfeeding experience.

There is sometimes confusion about what bonding is and what attachment is, and they're often used interchangeably (incorrectly). The way to look at it is to see each as one side of a coin. Bonding is the ongoing process of establishing the connection that a mother feels for her baby. It can be nearly instantaneous at birth when many women describe falling in love with their babies at first sight. It can also take time to feel that connection for many mothers, for whom the bonding process is unfolding over time. Both are equally valid. When mothers are dealing with perinatal mood and anxiety disorders they can feel disconnected and concerned about the impact this will have on bonding with their babies. Attachment is the view from the baby's side of the coin. This has to do with how secure and safe the baby feels in relationship with the caregiver/mother. Attachment is built on the interactions between baby and parents, and can be secure or insecure. Attachment is known to be stable over time, so the conditions that surrounded the formation of an attachment in early life will often play out in relationships later in life. The chapters in this Part will detail various aspects of bonding and attachment in the perinatal period.

CHAPTER 17

Bonding

Bonding had its introduction as a concept and a process back in 1976, with the publication of the book *Maternal-infant Bonding*, by Marshall Klaus[1] and John Kennell. The book was the first scientific exploration of the connection that forms after birth, and the effect that extended contact between mother and baby had on the quality of that attachment. As a direct result of this publication, hospitals all over the world began to reform their policies in favor of allowing mothers and babies to remain together for longer intervals immediately after birth. When my son Graham was born in a birth center in 1976, the buzzword of the day was bonding, and we "bonded" for an hour and a half with him continuously nursing at the breast. Everyone blessed this union, though I wouldn't recommend nursing all the time you are spending with your baby in close proximity. We were cemented together without question, a bond facilitated by the attitudes of staff surrounding me, who understood the importance of maternal attachment.

Several years later, the title of the book was revised to *Parent-Infant Bonding* (1982), demonstrating the wisdom of including the father, who is also forming an attachment to his child, with many interactive behaviors enhancing that connection. Another version has come out more recently called *Bonding: Building the Foundations of Secure Attachment and Independence* (Klaus, Kennel, & Klaus, 1996), with Phyllis Klaus joining these authors. A special connection between the mother and baby is hardwired into both through the rush of hormones that are coursing

---

1   When this book was about to be submitted for publication, I learned that Marshall Klaus died on August 15, 2017, at the age of 90. I had the privilege of meeting Marshall and Phyllis Klaus in 1985, and we became friends and colleagues. It is a sad loss for the world. Phyllis has written the Foreword to this book. Further down, I mention the loss of John Kennell too, who died in 2013.

through their bodies in those minutes and hours after birth. Forty years later, we know so much more about the dynamics of these hormones and the impact they have on the formation of this bond. Now you do too, after reading Part 2.

On a sad note, during the writing of this book, John Kennell passed away on August 27, 2013. He left behind an incredible legacy (along with Marshall Klaus) through the development of bonding theory and practice, and his research into the importance of doula care that reduces the level of interventions and improves the experience of mothers giving birth. He was one of the founders of Doulas of North America (DONA) in 1992, now an international organization for the promotion and training of doulas. Kennell was a wonderful advocate for mothers and babies, contributing to the field of pediatrics well into his late eighties. He will be missed. And now Marshall Klaus, who was his long-standing collaborator, has passed away too.

Prenatal Bonding

The formation of mothers' attachment their babies, called prenatal bonding, begins while they are still cradled within the body of their mothers. A pregnant woman who has been feeling the baby moving and kicking within her becomes sensitive to the intimate sensations that create a rhythm between the mother and unborn. She notices the patterns of movements that seem to begin just when she's ready to fall asleep. Some parents are known to spend time touching and talking to the bump, knowing that the being inside hears and feels the contact. All of these sensations and feelings are the ongoing communication of prenatal bonding. Although parents greet the baby for the first time after birth, the mother develops an ongoing relationship when the baby is felt moving inside, if not sooner.

Today, technology is creating new ways of bonding with the baby while it is still inside through the use of ultrasound scans, which can produce images in 3D and 4D (4D also includes the baby's movement). Once upon a time, when a woman went to see the health practitioner and listened to the baby's heartbeat, it was the primary way of connecting with the life she was carrying. When ultrasound fetascopes became the norm, it was possible to hear the heartbeat out loud, as opposed to an old-fashioned fetascope, in which only the practitioner could hear. If amniocentesis is done, and the sex is known, these parents can relate to their unborn baby specifically by sex, and often by name. It is now also possible to learn the sex of the baby through ultrasound, which enhances the prenatal bonding process. The use of prenatal ultrasound is often justified in terms of the bonding that parents feel through the image of the baby on the screen. What concerns me is how this reliance on an ultrasound image is superseding the physical and intimate connection a mother feels on the inside with her unborn child.

I believe that the UK has found the correct balance in the number of scans done during pregnancy, at two or three. There is a gross overindulgence in the U.S. in the number of scans done, especially for practices that have invested in ultrasound equipment for their offices. Those health care practitioners want to get their money's worth; they pay for their investment by using it. This isn't the case all the time when doctors refer mothers to radiologists or labs for this purpose. It can be seductive because it has the element of connecting parents to their babies while they're still inside, but the jury is still out on the long-range effects of the excess use of ultrasound. When it comes to prenatal bonding, the physical contact of body language speaks louder than monitoring devices and clinical tests, if women choose to listen. And there is no risk.

Communicating with the Preborn

The earlier a mother gets in touch with her baby, the better. Some mothers sing to their babies with tunes they'll sing again after birth. Some mothers meditate and feel a sense of communion with their unborn. An attunement through movements and rhythms is established as a mother and unborn are learning about each other during the creative process of life. Maternity-care professionals don't put much credibility in prenatal bonding, beyond what their technology can provide because few doctors can identify with the psychological needs of the mother. Their detached and rational, professional approach leaves most mothers feeling frustrated when they try to express the wonder and awe they feel about their unborn babies. Yet, with each day, she is gradually building an image of herself as a mother, reinforced by the regular movement of her baby, and developing an impression of her baby too.

electrochemical signals are transformed into meaningful messages, ideas, or memories cannot be explained in physical terms alone. The immature nervous system cannot account for the laying down of memories, and the transpersonal literature points to soul consciousness as an explanation of how the fetus receives input and translates these messages into memories.

Another leader of this consciousness movement is Wendy Anne McCarty, who wrote a book based on her work as a prenatal and perinatal psychologist called *Welcoming Consciousness: Supporting Babies' Wholeness from the Beginning of Life* (2012). She carries on the work that David Chamberlain and others began on early development and the stories that people tell about their journeys in the womb and during birth. She also explores the mysteries of our multidimensional selves from the baby's point of view through many case studies. In establishing an integrated model of early development, McCarty draws on the fundamental wisdom that "our primary nature is as conscious, sentient, non-physical beings that exist before and beyond physical human existence" (McCarty, 2012, p. 62).

An encyclopedic volume on consciousness before birth, and even before conception, was written by Elizabeth and Neil Carman called *Cosmic Cradle: Spiritual Dimensions of Life Before Birth* (2013). The Carmans traveled around the world meeting people, often children, who remember choosing to incarnate with specific parents, and shared memories of their time in the womb and their experiences as souls taking embodiment. There is a substantial section on prebirth communication between mothers and the spirits of their preconceived and gestating spirit-babies. There is also a detailed history of mystical traditions, in ancient and indigenous cultures across the globe, which honor incoming spirits. Here is an insightful comment from a preschooler who was an "old" soul: "There is more support for the incoming Soul if parents are welcoming, anticipating, and desiring. It's a more nourishing reception. The child gets off to a better start" (Carman & Carman, 2013, p. 189). *Cosmic Cradle* is a cornucopia of spiritual stories of life before birth.

Kelly Meehan is another gifted healer whose work involves the life of the soul before birth. She facilitates intuitive conversations in which the mother connects to the spirit of her baby through "soul baby communication," utilizing her prebirth communication soul cards and other empathic skills.

She works energetically with women experiencing cosmic pregnancies, and cosmic conceptions, working metaphysically with infertility, and empowering them to establish their connections to their spirit babies. She is a great advocate of women following their intuition so that they can experience the soul vibration of the incoming spirit. She has programs for cosmic pregnancy and cosmic conception and works privately with individuals who come for soul-baby counseling sessions, and integrative-energy therapy, which includes a good deal of bodywork. Kelly works with women from around the world who are committed to connecting with the spirit of their babies at an energetic-field level, establishing a bond before conception and during pregnancy. Her sessions create a sacred space for motherhood, full of heart and soul, tuning into the baby's soul and whatever her soul wants her to know (http://www.birthhealing.com/). Preconception consciousness is a growing field, with authors and practitioners who bring a truly spiritual dimension to the childbearing journey.

Bonding after Birth

Once babies are born, they need to be immediately returned to their mothers, whose body temperature is just right for babies when they are skin to skin, so long as there is a towel wrapped around them as the birth fluids dry on their skin. When an unmedicated baby is placed on the mother's abdomen and allowed to remain there without any interference, that baby will crawl up the mother's body and find the nipple of the breast with his or her mouth. As already discussed, it's the "breast crawl," and it is amazing to watch (YouTube has numerous videos of babies doing the breast crawl, and I included a clip of one in the last Part on breastfeeding).

Finding the breast is a reunion, a reconnection through nourishment and body contact that expands beyond the capacity to give and receive food. It is the comfort of a warm body and the sensual awareness of touch, taste, and smell. The familiar smell of the mother is what propels the baby up to the breast. This first meeting will be recreated every time the mother breastfeeds the baby. It is an embrace that transmits tenderness, joy, excitement, and apprehension for the family journey about to unfold. The days, months, and years ahead will extend the first moment into a pattern of love, and it is important to know that our beginning sets the tone for our future.

Bonding is the unspoken communication of attachment. Our first bond has an enormous bearing on how we continue to know love and experience attachment in life, and the way in which we make connections to others will reflect the level of integration we feel within ourselves. Before the publication of *Maternal-Infant Bonding* in 1976, bonding was not a concern in the maternity units of North America, where mother and baby were routinely separated and isolated at opposite ends of the hospital floor. The amount of time that the mother and infant spent together was limited to feedings, more often than not, with plastic bottles and teats. Babies imprinted to the detached handling of nursing staff instead of the loving arms of their mothers.

In other industrialized countries, mothers and babies were kept together in hospitals, and separation was a mostly American phenomenon. Times have changed, as we now know there are so many critical biological requirements happening after birth, and we continue to learn more year after year. Attitudes, behaviors, and policies have changed dramatically in the last several decades.

We know that one of the crucial benefits of birth stress, initiated by an abundance of ACTH and adrenaline within the fetus, is the activation in the newborn of a hormonal condition essential to the physical formation of bonding (Condon et al., 2004; Gao et al., 2015; Polettini et al., 2015).

Some Useful Articles

http://www.drmomma.org/2008/01/fetal-lungs-protein-release-triggers.html

http://www.sciencedaily.com/releases/2015/06/150622162023.htm

http://www.sciencedaily.com/releases/2015/10/151026132136.htm?utm_source=feedburner&utm_medium=email&utm_campaign=Feed%3A+sciencedaily%2Fhealth_medicine%2Fpregnancy_and_chil dbirth+%28Pregnancy+and+Childbirth+News+--+ScienceDaily%29

This biological preparation for reconnecting with our mothers is counterbalanced by what Klaus and Kennell called the "maternal sensitive period," also hormonally induced, wherein the mother is programmed particularly by endorphins and oxytocin to receive her child. The hormones secreted during the birth process in both the mother and infant are in abundance during the first hour after birth, bearing physiological authenticity to the sensitive period for bonding. The rhythm of this reunion is a delicate attunement, biologically hardwired, and leaving an everlasting imprint, so long as nothing disturbs the hormonal balance that primes the meeting when conditions are optimal.

The dynamic between parents and infant is unique, and the attachment bespeaks a union that will endure over time. We have specific bonds to many people in life, but none as important as that with our mother, and all subsequent connections to others will depend on this first attachment. The development of our sense of self will evolve from the primary relationships we know as infants. The energy that holds the universe together, and the basic intelligence of all things created, is love. As our babies are born, the best way to receive them is through deep and expressed love, a journey to the heart, which satisfies the need to give and receive love. The breast crawl, where the newly born infant will crawl up the mother's abdomen to the breast and latch on, is the quintessential journey to the heart.

Skin-to-Skin Contact

If nature is allowed to prevail during birth, then the baby would stay naked on the mother's body after it had made that primal journey up the body to find the breast, and the mother and baby would be wrapped together while skin to skin. We know about the importance of skin-to-skin contact between a mother and baby, and the regulating effects that it has; it stabilizes the baby's temperature better than any machine could, it normalizes heart and breathing rates, it reduces stress hormone production, and blood sugar stabilizes too (https://babygooroo.com/articles/10-benefits-of-skin-to-skin-contact).

There is a plethora of research on how the baby's skin and gut are colonized by the mother's bacteria, offering protection from pathogens and allergies, and referred to as the microbiome (Harman & Wakeford, 2016). These protective factors are part of the reason why kangaroo care is so beneficial to premature babies, who grow and develop at a much faster rate when held close to the body. Rather than being separated by an incubator that restricts the level of touch that is possible, the baby is positioned on the mother's chest, touching the skin, and the father/partner, if around. Kangaroo care is a metaphor for keeping the baby as close as a kangaroo

Physiologic Birth

In a recent consensus statement by three North American midwifery organizations in support of physiologic childbirth, the connection between a normal birth and bonding was revealed (Supporting Healthy and Normal Physiologic Childbirth: A Consensus Statement by ACNM, MANA, and NACPM, 2013).

> Research … confirms how critical it is to foster a supportive environment for women and newborns through birth and the postpartum period," said MANA (Midwives Alliance North America) Executive Director Geraldine Simkins, CNM, MSN. "The foundation of social and emotional competence is shaped by the interactions newborns have with their mothers, and evidence suggests that normal physiological birth plays a role in healthy mother-infant attachment (U.S. Midwifery Organizations Make the Case for Normal Physiologic Birth, June 5, 2012).

Once the baby is born, women need a supportive environment to continue after they are discharged from the hospital. This is in short supply in English-speaking cultures like the U.S. and UK. The Netherlands is one society that has taken the postnatal adjustments of mothers seriously. Someone comes to the home on a daily basis to help the mother manage the new demands on her time. The purpose and value of this support are to facilitate the bond between parents and child, while other household responsibilities are being taken care of by someone else. A postpartum doula provides this kind of care, but for a price. I talked about postpartum doulas earlier in Part 1, in the discussion about matrescence, and how support allows matrescence to unfold naturally. As continuing research demonstrates the interconnections between child development and bonding, it becomes imperative to normalize physiologic birth and provide the resources for new mothers that enhance the bonding process and the attachment we form with our children.

In January 2015, Childbirth Connection, the American non-profit organization that works to improve the quality of maternity care, published the report authored by Sarah J Buckley, MD on *Hormonal Physiology of Childbearing: Evidence and Implications for Women, Babies and Maternity*

Care. Childbirth Connection is now part of the National Partnership for Women and Families. It was formerly known as the Maternity Center Association, founded in 1918 to improve the maternal and infant mortality rates, and train midwives in New York City. I gave birth to my second child in their Childbearing Center, the first birth center to open in the U.S. (1975), in a beautiful brownstone on the Upper East Side of Manhattan. Buckley's report is a much-needed antidote to medicalized childbirth, with its cascade of interventions that can disrupt natural biological processes. It documents the practices for promoting, supporting, and protecting true physiological childbirth. The report highlights the importance of the physiological onset of labor and then examines the major endogenous hormonal systems that are key to the perinatal period, and the maternity-care practices that interfere. The positive aspects are:

> ... physiologic childbearing facilitates beneficial outcomes in women and babies by promoting fetal readiness for birth and safety during labor, enhancing labor effective- ness, providing physiologic help with labor stress and pain, promoting maternal and newborn transitions and maternal adaptations, and optimizing breastfeeding and maternal-infant attachment, among many processes (p. 1, Executive Summary).

Successful lactation and bonding are hormonally mediated processes that are intertwined with the biologic processes of childbirth. This means that disruption of perinatal hormonal physiology may impact not only labor and delivery but also breastfeeding and maternal-infant attachment. A birth that occurs in harmony with the hormonal and physiological processes provides optimum experiences for the mother and baby. This report is the new evidence-base for best practice in maternity care that allows birth to happen spontaneously, respectful of how natural biological rhythms regulate the stress response while opening the heart for the mother/baby dyad to receive each other after a sacred journey.

CHAPTER 18

Attachment Theory

The origins of attachment theory began in the mid-20th century when John Bowlby initiated studies in England investigating how attachment to a primary caregiver is a biological requirement for the survival of the species. Bowlby's belief that human beings need a secure attachment relationship was based on his early studies on the adverse effects of "maternal deprivation." He recognized that separation from the mother in early childhood impacted on personality development, and that mental health depends on the quality of parental care in the earliest years of life. He felt it was essential "that the infant and young child should experience a warm, intimate, and continuous relationship with his mother (or permanent mother substitute) in which both find satisfaction and enjoyment" (Bowlby, 1952, p. 11). The absence of this kind of connection is what he called maternal deprivation, and much of the early research he conducted was with homeless children or those who were confined to orphanages, hospitals, or other institutions. Under those circumstances, no one person cared for the infant/child in a personal way or with whom this child felt secure. Many of these children suffered from failure to thrive due to the lack of this kind of personal attention, and those who survived this state of affairs often experienced mental illness. Bowlby went on to write a classic trilogy called *Attachment and Loss*, with three volumes that covered *Attachment* (Vol. 1), *Separation* (Vol. 2), and *Loss* (Vol. 3).

Mary Ainsworth, Bowlby's American counterpart, expanded attachment theory with her empirical studies of The Strange Situation. This was an experimental situation (laboratory playroom) designed to test the security of attachment between the mother and child (who was 12 to 18 months old). First, they play together, and then an unfamiliar woman joins them, and then the mother leaves the room, leaving the child to play with this

Attachment theory recognizes four components of attachment: 1) a safe haven, 2) a secure base, 3) proximity seeking, and 4) separation protest (or distress). A safe haven is a caregiver who a distressed child can return to for comfort and soothing when aroused or threatened. A reliable caregiver is also the secure base from which the child can move out into the world to explore. When the base is unresponsive or unreliable, exploration is inhibited and so is the expression of needs. Proximity seeking is triggered when the infant experiences stress and seeks security and safety within the orbit of that caregiver. Separation protest (distress/anxiety) indicates how the child becomes upset and distressed when separated from the caregiver. When we create a secure environment for our children, we foster a secure attachment that is the cornerstone of healthy infant development, as well as a secure base from which the baby can explore, learn, and develop life skills.

Optimal development occurs in an environment of safety in which emotional synchrony and resonance between an infant and caregiver/mother take place. Mutually eliciting responses can be observed between the caregiver and the baby during the newborn period, and babies can mimic their mothers or fathers in the early days. There is another kind of synchrony observed (in slow motion) during the newborn period, illustrating how babies move their bodies in response to caregivers' speech in a finely tuned dance of maternal/infant mutuality. This coordinated interaction is the beginning of social responsiveness and demonstrates how attuned the mother/baby dyad is. "Serve and return" interactions happen like conversational turn-taking, proto-conversational, as each elicits a response from the other in similar ways to a conversation using language: in this case, body language. Social intelligence will grow from these first synchronized communications that wire the brain for interpersonal connection, and also lay the foundation for the kind of open responsiveness required for committed relationships later in life.

The Neuroscience of Attachment

In the 45 years since Ainsworth was conducting her experiments, an extensive body of research in the areas of neuroscience, psychology, and infant development has contributed to the enormous expansion of the theory. The neuroscience behind attachment reveals some of the mysteries of the instinctive interactions between a mother and baby, demonstrating how the infant's brain responds to attachment behaviors, as well as the effects of stress and health on brain development. This data confirms Bowlby's comprehensive theory. We know that from the end of pregnancy through the second year of life, sometimes called the 1001 Days (or part of it), the human brain goes through an accelerated period of growth. This early proliferation consumes more energy than any other stage in life and requires adequate nutrition and interpersonal experiences for optimal maturation.

The emphasis is on the development of the right brain, which is deeply connected to the sympathetic and parasympathetic nervous systems. It controls essential functions that support survival and coping, along with the limbic system, which is the neurological seat of emotions. The limbic system is where the hippocampus and amygdala structures are linked to memory and emotional regulation. Babies lack the skills to regulate the intensity or duration of emotions, leaving them incapable of maintaining a state of equilibrium on their own. It is the reliable and devoted relationship with the mother (or another caring person) that supports this emotional equilibrium until the baby develops the ability to self-regulate. The baby relies on the attuned relationship with a caregiver to offset any dysregulation created by stress, and stress to a baby can be anything new and different. While healthy attachment promotes optimal brain development, stress and trauma can impair it.

Reflective functioning is a uniquely human capacity that enables perspective-taking while monitoring the actions of ourselves and others. Sometimes called "mind-mindedness," it allows the parents to understand their babies' behavior regarding their internal states, such as intentions, beliefs, feelings, and desires. When parents experience their baby as an intentional being, the child develops an understanding of the mental states of others, and how to regulate their own internal experiences. The parents' capacity for reflective functioning helps the infant begin to make sense of primary feeling states by appropriate responsiveness communicating to the child their understanding of the child's inner states. Reflective functioning is an emotional process that allows us to engage emotionally with another person, providing a sense of security from feeling known. In any relationship, reflective functioning means we are cognitively and emotionally online for another person, and cognitively and emotionally available.

Mirror Neurons

A group of Italian neuroscientists, doing animal research in the mid-1990s, discovered *mirror neurons* (nerve cells) that work on the basis that the perception (by a monkey) of some action in another (the scientist) will cause the motor area of the brain to activate in the monkey. The experiment demonstrated a link between the perceptual and motor areas of the brain, and that a single neuron had both perceptual and motor capabilities. In an interview with Daniel Siegel, MD, he explained how they work: "To say it simply: they let you imitate an intentional action" (The Mindful Practitioner, webinar series, NICABM, 2011). The brain is always creating maps composed of clusters of neural firing, and mirror neurons are mapping the intentional state of another. Siegel says: "The absolutely revolutionary finding here is that these researchers were able to illuminate the way neural firing maps create symbolic neural firing patterns that are mapping out mental states" (Siegel, 2011). The prefrontal cortex in the brain makes a map of the mind of another person. Mirror neurons are involved in the imitation of action and simulate internal states, which is the root of empathy. The way that this plays out is my mirror neurons can pick up your internal state, which triggers the same state in me, and this informs me of how you are feeling. This is empathic imagination.

Another way of understanding this is the physiology of empathy, and it's also the neurobiology of "we." Siegel's interpersonal neurobiology explains how people get close to each other because they can (below conscious awareness) sense that their neuro-signals are inside the other person. Mirror neurons are the neurological substrates for the process of mirroring when we reflect to the other person what we are sensing from them. During reflective functioning, marked mirroring is an extension of mirroring that helps babies understand what they are feeling by punctuating the interaction with reassuring expressions from the parent, often in the form of facial expressions and voice tone. This marking helps the baby know the feelings belong to him; the parent understands, and the baby learns how to manage his emotions. Marked mirroring hands the baby's experience back to her, framing it for her, and making it coherent and explicit.

Resonance Circuits

There is a neural circuit in the brain called the insula that connects the mirror neurons and the limbic areas of the brain, and sends signals to the brainstem and the body and back up to the middle prefrontal areas, and this set of circuits is how we resonate physiologically with others. These resonance circuits create a pathway that connects us to one another. They also offer an explanation for emotional contagion, which we talked about in Part 2 (Hormones) when stress interferes with the flow of oxytocin because other people in the room are expressing fear or anxiety.

We know that there are neural circuits around the heart and the body that are interwoven with the resonance circuits of the brain. The experience of "feeling felt" helps us develop the internal strength of self-regulation. Initially, the responsive parent helps to regulate babies' emotions by responding to their cues for help when they cry. With time, the secure baby can internalize the ability to self-soothe and establish relationships that build resilience and safety. Siegel has been at the forefront of research into the neural mechanisms of attachment and his findings support much of the previous research.

> Although the attachment researchers did not study the brain directly, these overall outcomes parallel our middle prefrontal functions in many ways: securely attached children developed good bodily regulation, attunement to others, emotional balance, response flexibility, fear modulation, empathy and insight, and moral awareness ... From the viewpoint of interpersonal neurobiology, this strongly suggests that secure parent-child interactions promote the growth of the integrative fibers of the middle prefrontal region of the child's brain (Siegel, 2010, p. 170).

Siegel tells us that the resonance circuitry that allows us to feel felt and connect to one another also helps to regulate our internal state. He describes the "window of tolerance" as the band of arousal within which we can function well. When we widen that window, we can maintain a state of equilibrium when faced with stresses that generally would knock us off our center. A narrow window of tolerance can leave us feeling constricted in our lives. When we are within our window of tolerance, we stay receptive. When we

Couples learn to feel with and for others, to recognize what Johnson calls "the ancient code of attachment" that each partner brings to the relationship, repairs any toxic damage that surfaces when we are stressed, as we reach out to the other, knowing there will be a response. This is called "effective dependency" because emotional isolation is the enemy of humankind, no matter how independent we believe we are. The paradox is that effective dependency helps us grow into stronger people. These healthy models make it safe for partners to ask "are you there for me?" Sue Johnson also explains how trauma can be healed when a person can seek comfort in the arms of another. I will discuss the adult attachment bond again in Part 5.

CHAPTER 19

Attachment Parenting

Attachment parenting is an approach to parenting that fosters a secure attachment, trust, empathy, affection, and healthy development for children through responsive interactions. For parents, it offers the gift of love, confidence, and a deep connection that lasts a lifetime. It encourages parents to be "good enough" parents, not to strive for perfection. An essential tenet of attachment parenting is respect for children and their needs. It is the empathetic response to those needs that begins the pattern for future relationships and as just mentioned, for the internal capacity of the child's self-regulation. Attachment parenting is often associated with certain practices, such as babywearing, co-sleeping/bedsharing, breastfeeding, and baby-led weaning. But these practices are enhancements to attachment parenting, and the focus is on the development of the baby/parent dyad. The bottom line in attachment parenting is love *writ large,* that transcends our own childhood experiences, our pasts, and moves us out into the community to effect positive change.

Attachment Parenting International (API) defines their mission: "to educate and support all parents in raising secure, joyful, and empathic children to strengthen families and create a more compassionate world." This resonates with the section below "a new generation of peacemakers," and our need to raise children with kindness, respect, and dignity, "and to model, in our interactions with them, the way we'd like them to interact with others." It's the antidote to emotionally and behaviorally troubled youth who lack a secure and healthy attachment to a parent or primary caregiver.

API offers a parent education program that includes a comprehensive series of classes for every stage and age of child development, helping parents feel confident in developing a nurturing, connected relationship with their children. They continue to support parents with groups, online support, and publications. They have synthesized research from psychology, child development, and neuroscience focused on the behaviors and outcomes of attachment theory for over 60 years and applied this knowledge to everyday parenting practices so that parents regain trust in their intuition as they grow as a family.

The provocative front cover of the May 21, 2012 issue of *Time Magazine*, which shows a fit mother breastfeeding (standing up) her 3-year-old child standing on a chair to reach the breast, created quite a stir. The title of the article "Are You Mom Enough?" (Pickert, 2012) generated numerous responses about attachment parenting, including one by Jessica Kramer, with another provocative title: "The Woman On the Cover is Both Madonna and Whore."

In her article, Kramer emphasizes the disrespectful attitude towards women who are already struggling to give birth normally in an environment that is overwhelmingly medicalized, and *Time's* incendiary article only increases the pressure to perform in a certain way. Mothers in the *Time* article get the short end of the stick, but William Sears, MD, the founder of the Attachment Parenting movement, is given much more credence. He sounds sane while the mothers sound extreme. The brouhaha around this *Time* piece, and which Kramer picks up on and uses in her title, is the cultural split between mother and sexual being. Mothers are not supposed to be sexy, and sexy women are not maternal. The woman on the cover is both, and that is enormously threatening to the status quo. This echoes what I said in the last Part about the tension between cultural and biological femininity.

What Is It?

Attachment parenting (AP) is a highly intuitive, high-touch style of parenting that encourages a strong early attachment and advocates consistent parental responsiveness to babies' dependency needs. Instead of delivering a prescription for when to breastfeed or when to respond to a cry, attachment parenting encourages parents to learn and work with their baby's particular cues. It is a deep attunement that defies any one-size-fits-all approach to parenting. William Sears and his wife Martha, both medical professionals, wrote the groundbreaking book for the movement: *The*

Attachment Parenting Book (2001). Their book articulates the benefits of attachment parenting for both parent and child, and explains how AP improves development, makes discipline easier, and even promotes independence (which many might find counterintuitive). Additional topics include AP for working parents, attachment fathering, weaning your child from AP, as well as the science behind why attachment parenting works. The authors' intention in writing the book was to offset the years of advice that was discussed earlier (in Chapter 3 of The Fourth Trimester) about not spoiling children with too much loving attention. Here's what they say: "… this book is our attempt to give back to parents the instinctual, high-touch way of caring for their children that decades of *detachment advice* have robbed them of" (emphasis mine; Sears & Sears, 2001, p. ix). The book offers valuable guidance and reassurance to families choosing to parent consciously and sensitively. The movement that grew out of this approach to parenting is a 21st century phenomenon, and it appeared after the days when I was working with new mothers on an ongoing basis. No one sits on the fence with this movement; you either subscribe to the style or you refute it with vehemence. The polarization on this issue is a reflection of the general polarization around birth and related matters. There needs to be a middle way.

The 7 Baby Bs

The core elements of *The Attachment Parenting Book* are the **7 Baby Bs of Attachment Parenting**:

1. **Birth/bonding.** This is the substance of what this Part you are reading now is about, including skin-to-skin contact, the baby's quiet alert state at birth, touch, eye contact, and talking. Babies recognize their parents' voices, delaying routine procedures, breastfeeding in the first hour, and privacy.

2. **Breastfeeding.** Part 3 of this book covers this section.

3. **Babywearing.** They discuss different holds: clutch (for nursing on the side), cradle (horizontal), or snuggle (vertical), the benefits to vestibular control and other internal systems, and wearing the baby down to sleep.

4. **B**edsharing. This is attachment parenting at night; the mother and baby sleep better (with some exceptions for mothers who are hypersensitive to baby noises), breastfeeding is easier, safety in co-sleeping, weaning from nighttime AP.

5. **B**elief in the baby's cries. Crying is a signal, not a manipulation, learning the cues of the baby's communication, damage caused by crying it out (elevated stress hormones), and a great little quote: "if you listen to them when they're young, they'll listen to you when they're older" (Sears & Sears, 2001, p. 82).

6. **B**alance and boundaries. Boundary setting, what the baby needs most is a happy mother, manage resentment by changing the cause of it, enmeshment, baby breaks and avoiding burnout, rest, and working as a team with a partner.

7. **B**eware of baby trainers. A one-size-fits-all approach with no research supporting it, baby training (see below) promotes insensitivity and is based on a misperception of the parent/child relationship, causes shut-down syndrome, and trust is lost.

The 11 Commandments for Balanced Attachment Parenting

Though it isn't always recognized, attachment parenting seeks balance in how parenting unfolds. Here are the 11 Commandments for Balanced Attachment Parenting:

1. Thou shalt take care of thyself.

2. Thou shalt honor thy husband/**partner** [my inclusive term added] with his share of the attachment parenting.

3. Thou shalt avoid the prophets of bad baby advice.

4. Thou shalt surround thyself with helpful and supportive friends.

5. Thou shalt have help at home.

6. Thou shalt get to know thy baby.

7. Thou shalt give children what they need, not what they want.

8. Thou shalt sleep when the baby sleeps.

9. Thou shalt groom and adorn thyself.

10. Thou shalt heal thy past.

11. Thou shalt realize thou art not perfect.

Attachment parenting is about being responsive to your baby's cues. I wonder if it were called *"responsive parenting,"* whether it would generate the kind of hysterical reaction that it often does. Being responsive is vital to babies' needs, and it engenders trust inside babies when they know that their needs will be met. Trust is an essential first stage in psychosocial development as defined by Erik Erikson in the 20th century. Being attached seems to produce a critical stance, and that is probably because of generations of detachment parenting in the last century. The intent of the Sears' in writing their book is to turn the tide of such insensitive parenting and help parents re-find their instincts. This is also one of my intentions for writing this book.

The Blossom Method™

While I was writing this book, I discovered another one that illustrates ways to interact with your baby by learning the many ways he or she communicates using its tongue, facial expressions, and body (Sabel, 2012). This is the essence of nonverbal communication at the very start of life. The author, Vivien Sabel, grew up with a deaf mother and learned how to read the subtlest cues in body language to understand her mother and communicate without words. The Blossom Method™ uses a three-step approach that expands on the mirror neuron phenomenon we discussed earlier in Chapter 18. The three steps are to observe, mirror, and respond. Observation involves noticing the movements of the tongue, mouth, and lips in particular, and other body language that reveals what the baby needs. Mirroring what you have observed shows the baby that you "heard" what was "said." Responding offers reassurance that you understand what was communicated and both of you are part of a two-way dialogue. By following the baby's lead, you are learning his or her language. I have worked with babies for more than 20 years and did not know just how much information can be gleaned by what the tongue is doing. Tongue talking is the way that babies make requests of their parents and offer information about what they are experiencing.

The **hungry tongue** can be observed as two different movements: an "O" shape, and a tongue that moves in and out of the mouth. There's the **searching tongue** that moves from side to side, and this is often accompanied by eye-scanning. The windy (gassy) tongue/facial expression involves a flaccid but full bottom lip and an appearance of fullness. There's even a tongue move for the body's elimination, and this has a pointed, sharp-looking shape that extends out of the mouth fully. This is usually accompanied by other signs, such as a strained smile, wincing, a look of discomfort, an arched back, and a tight stomach.

The book is full of other body signs that you can learn to read as you "listen" with your eyes in this wonderful way of nonverbally parenting your baby. Sabel says, "Conversing with our baby from such an early age will help her to feel and experience trust and to develop confidence in her relationships with you and others. If your baby feels understood, contained, and seen (and therefore heard), this will give her strong foundations for her emotional and physical development" (Sabel, 2012, pp. 40-41). I have been so impressed by this book that I highly recommend that you purchase it. It exemplifies all the responsive parenting that this chapter is about. Vivien Sabel and I have become friends and colleagues who share a vision for enhancing the connections within the mother-baby dyad and the healthy development of attachment in families.

CHAPTER 20

Going Against the Grain

Behavior-Based Techniques (aka Baby Training)

The antithesis of attachment is baby training, also called sleep training. The queen of this approach to childrearing is Gina Ford, a nurse who never had children herself, who we first met in Chapter 3, in The Fourth Trimester. I had to force myself to read this book, even though I disagreed with so much of it, to understand why so many parents would choose to go down this route. It seems to appeal to people who are accustomed to establishing a level of order in their lives and want to be able to maintain this state after the baby arrives. This fails to recognize the fundamental changes in your life that are created when a baby comes into the picture. "Getting back to normal" is the driving force when normal has changed so dramatically. Why does the baby have to pay such a terrible price for "the secret to calm and confident parenting" (the book's subtitle)? It goes against the grain of mothers finding and trusting their instincts in how they parent and instead, institutes a regimen so precise, it would be better suited to the military. The baby wouldn't have read the instructions.

As I said earlier, it imposes serious pressures on the mother to conform to a prescriptive routine that becomes more imperative than sensitivity to the baby's needs and cues. Here's what she says about slings: "Very small babies are also inclined to go straight to sleep the minute you hold them close to your chest [duh!], which defeats the whole purpose of my routines" (Ford, 2006, pp. 15-16, comment added). In her own words, she is doing what is so prevalent in birth and parenting, thinking she can improve on what nature had intended.

Gina Ford has never been awash in those hormonal cocktails that we've been talking about and has no idea how it feels to be a postpartum woman adjusting to changes on so many levels. Her assertion that babies at birth should be able to go three hours between feeds is wrong and is a set up for failure. Breastfeeding newborn babies usually can manage about two hours. Her instructions for expressing milk using pumps is far too dependent on machines and probably will be bad conditioning since milk that should be going to the baby is going into bottles instead, and pumps do not have the same effect on the breasts as nursing. There are remnants of John Watson (Chapter 3) and his detached style of parenting in her comment: "do not overhandle his small body and exhaust him ... when cuddling him during the wind-down time, do not talk and avoid eye contact, as it can overstimulate him and result in him becoming overtired and not settling" (Ford, p. 115; babies are always male in her book), and this prohibition is repeated throughout the book.

We just read in Daniel Siegel's Facebook post how the Still Face experiment can interfere with a baby's need for attunement. Ford's directions invite a disturbance to the physiological equilibrium that the baby requires. Her idea of preparation for birth is to accumulate all the baby paraphernalia you'll need in advance. She also mentions "lots of recent research" many times without providing any references. Her "milk feeding chart for the first year" (p. 131) is an exercise in precision that no baby ever knew. I guess for people who want to be directed on how to parent on a blow-by-blow basis, this book is it. My overall reaction after reading over 300 pages of dire recommendations is "UGH!"

The Impact on the Baby and the Mother

Why is this a problem? Because we now understand what the consequences are of letting a baby cry for a long time (even 10 to 12 minutes that Ford admits to). It creates a chain of internal reactions that include a cycle of hyperarousal and dissociation from the distress that the baby feels. *Hyperarousal* comes from the engagement of the sympathetic nervous system, increasing the baby's heart rate, blood pressure, and breathing rate, and the baby's expression of this state of distress is crying. Crying is a signal that will progress to screaming if there is no response. Major stress hormones are secreted, which causes a hypermetabolic state in the developing brain. Prolonged periods spent in this state are damaging and can cause increased levels of thyroid hormones and vasopressin, which are triggered in response to an unsafe and challenging environment. Vasopressin is also linked to nausea and vomiting, and explains as to why some babies vomit after extended crying.

The second part of the cycle is *dissociation*, when the baby disengages from the external world and retreats into an internal state marked by numbing, avoidance, compliance, and non-reaction. It's a form of resignation, where the baby feels hopeless and helpless to affect its environment.

> The infant tries to repair the disequilibrium and misattunement but cannot, and so disengages, becomes inhibited, and strives to avoid attention, to become "unseen." This metabolic shutting-down is a passive state in response to an unbearable situation, and is the opposite of hyperarousal…In this state, pain-numbing endogenous opiates and behavior-inhibiting stress hormones, such as cortisol, are elevated. Blood pressure decreases, as does the heart rate, despite the still-circulating adrenaline (Porter, 2009).

The baby now needs to rally all its resources for survival and to maintain homeostasis, rather than for learning and developing.

In Lauren Lindsey Porter's elegant article on "The Science of Attachment: Biological Roots of Love," she explains that when babies are distressed, there are biochemical changes in the right brain that have long-term effects. In the baby, states become traits, meaning that these states of hyperarousal and dissociation become part of the personality structure that is forming because they are happening when the brain is at its maximum vulnerability. When this is a chronic situation, it can cause impaired brain development and atrophy.

Sleep training puts babies into this cycle of hyperarousal and dissociation, potentially damaging their development. "To think that since the infant has passively accepted the new sleep system, the sleep training is thus 'successful,' is to misunderstand the workings of the infant brain" (Porter, 2009). Go back and reread the Neuroscience of Attachment section in Chapter 18 to understand how this disrupts the organization of the prefrontal cortex.

CHAPTER 21

Partners and Peace

Father's/Partner's Attachment

When we talked about skin-to-skin contact in Chapter 17, I mentioned the importance of fathers and partners to this precious connection. Although the mother-baby dyad holds primacy over others based on its psychobiological underpinnings, the baby is cultivating "affectional bonds" within other non-maternal relationships too. Through skin-to-skin contact, the father is attuning to his baby, and the baby is absorbing new information from another source of love. As the baby grows, the father becomes a more central figure, and his role evolves as another secure base from which the child ventures out into the world. The baby is supported by a variety of relationships that influence growth and development, including siblings and other relatives, but the other parent is the most significant one beyond the mother.

There are several activities that a father can engage in with his baby: diaper/nappy changing is not the most pleasant one, but it offers opportunities to communicate in many ways, including the Blossom Method™. Fathers/partners can hold, caress, and carry (babywearing) the baby. Bathing was a favorite in our house: my children's father was the bath master in our home. Playing, reading, or singing can also be effective. I recently saw a Facebook video of a father, whose crying baby was strapped into a carrier, who sang a song with his guitar and the baby was asleep in minutes. Even bottle-feeding, hopefully with breast milk, is a way for fathers to interact on an intimate basis with their babies.

All of these activities are fostering the attachment between the baby and father/partner, cementing the bond of love. The father need not feel left out or incompetent in caring for his baby. He needs to define how he wants to interact and invest some time in the effort to do so. Sometimes mothers feel that they are the only ones who know how to do it right and can be exclusive. Fathers need to assert their right to learn how so they can also engage in babycare as well. In this way, the father is attuning to his baby and becoming an essential part of the parental connection that the baby needs for optimal growth and development.

Parental Investment

The more a father invests in his attachment to his children, the healthier and stronger the child will be in moving out into the world. He becomes a positive role model for loving care that expands on the mother's role of nurturing and nourishment. We saw how, in Part 2, the father also has some hormonal changes at the end of pregnancy and in the early days of parenting. These foster his experience of connecting with his baby as he transforms into a father. With more fathers taking an active role in the growth and development of their children, evolutionary cultural changes will make the old way of remote fathering obsolete. Children will grow up with a much more solid foundation that empowers them to meet the challenges that life presents with resilience and equanimity. Also, mothers will benefit from the sharing of the load, which can only be good for the relationship. When I created The Birth Empowerment Workshop in 1988, it was to help couples find their way to an empowered birth and parenting experience while remaining lovers on the journey to parenthood. Here are some of the fathers' testimonials:

> As a father, I feel calm and self-assured in unspecific ways. The workshop added to those feelings.

> I wonder if I would now be taking such an active role in the care of our Baby. The workshop helped teach me how a father can participate with daily care. It reinforced the feeling of excitement vs. anxiety.

Attached fatherhood will make a big difference in how the next generation of children experience and share intimacy, grounded in a felt experience from both parents at the start of life.

A New Generation of Peacemakers

There is no question that babies who are well-attached become better lovers later on in life. I'm not just talking about how they make love. I'm talking about how they express love for others at all levels: intimate, family, social, parental, and most important, unconditional love. It makes sense that generations of people who were raised on the limited attachment, or the detachment approach to parenting, are going to feel challenged by intimacy. We want it, but it can feel threatening when we have so little experience with it. If anything, we have learned to push it away, unintentionally.

When we have a secure and intimate attachment, our capacity to be loving and sharing with another is easy and natural. The more encouragement we can give for positive attachment experiences, the more our children will grow up to be at peace with themselves and others. Fostering the connection between parent and child, and between parents, is the first step in creating a new generation of peacemakers. An excellent book on this subject was written by Marcy Axness, called *Parenting for Peace: Raising the Next Generation of Peacemakers* (2012). Her seven foundational principles for effective, healthy, and joyful parenting spell PARENTS:

1. (**P**)resence – being fully engaged, right here, right now

2. (**A**)wareness – the knowledge to be effective

3. (**R**)hythm – a fundamental human pacing need

4. (**E**)xample – the ultimate mode of teaching and learning

5. (**N**)urturance – the practical demonstration of love

6. (**T**)rust – calm reliance upon processes outside your control

7. (**S**)implicity – the absence of complication and excess (which happens to be a big part of my message as well – SIMPLIFY!)

In addition to the seven principles, Axness takes the reader through seven steps on the developmental road to raising peaceful individuals. **Step One:** *Pro-Growth Choices – Cultivating a Fertile Mind and Body* is about getting ready for pregnancy. **Step Two:** *Attuned Conception – a Quantum Collaboration* details the significance of the first moments around conscious conception. **Step Three:** *Radiant Pregnancy – Harnessing the Power of the Womb* is a sensitive examination of pregnancy from the mother and baby's experiences. **Step Four:** *Empowered Birth – The Ultimate First Impression* discusses the many elements of how birth is conducted and the value of giving birth powerfully. **Step Five:** *Nature's Peace Plan – Installing Peacemaker Hardware in Year One* is where you are at this moment. It includes much of what we have been discussing about bonding and attachment, and consists of the neurobiology of the first year of life. **Step Six:** *The Enchanted Years – Toddlers through Kindergarten: Playing, Puttering, and Peace* describes how children learn, and it brought Rudolf Steiner's Waldorf education system to life for me. **Step Seven:** *Shepherd Them into the World – Shaping and Sharing Peace* is about childhood and the many challenges it presents when raising children to be sensitive and peaceful individuals. At the end of each chapter, she applies the seven principles in a way that integrates the processes with the material.

Interference and Facilitation

In the book, Axness draws our attention to how epidurals can impact on the attachment process. She explains: "25 percent of babies born with epidurals have difficulty in quickly, easily and smoothly latching on for breastfeeding; and *epidurals partially interfere with the release of oxytocin that normally occurs at birth,* which can affect bonding and the mother's falling-in-love feelings for her baby" (emphasis mine; Axness, 2012, p. 142). That is a significant outcome of obstetric anesthesia and could be an explanation for why some mothers get off to a bumpy start with breastfeeding. We are just starting to realize the impact it has on the development of a strong bond between the mother and baby. This is rarely talked about by birthcare practitioners as a possible side effect of epidural when they are advising about the common side effects of anesthesia (assuming this is done appropriately) as part of informed consent. It may appear in the literature, but not in the birthing room. Reading this during the postnatal period doesn't help you if you have had this experience, I know. However, it can contribute to your choices when you give birth in the future. If you are still pregnant when you read this, you have more information to consider when thinking about pain relief during labor and delivery.

Axness also explains how a secure relationship is the ground upon which the orbitofrontal cortex (OFC) in the brain develops. This part of the brain is a region within the prefrontal cortex of the frontal lobe that Siegel describes above, and was mentioned in the attachment-theory section. The OFC is the regulating and integrating structure of the brain that nurtures social and emotional intelligence. This becomes internalized as self-regulation and includes our ability to modulate moods, emotions, reactions, and sensory processing.

The OFC is fundamental to the development of skills for peace and for being human with other humans. This part of the brain is also involved in sensemaking and decision making. The OFC is critical for adaptive learning. It is also the seat of autobiographical memory and recall. The circuitry wires up in direct response to the quality of the primary attachment relationships. The nourishment for the OFC is empathy, connection, and presence. As Axness says:

> *Parenting for Peace* details a unique seven-step, seven-principle roadmap for hardwiring our babies and children with the brain circuitry for such essential peacemaker capacities as self-regulation, empathy, intelligence, trust, and imagination. The win-win is that a child wired in this vibrantly healthy way is a joy to parent, and as an adult has the heart to embrace and exemplify peace, the mind to innovate solutions to social and ecological challenges, and the will to enact them. To be successful in a changing world.
>
> [The book] offers readers a welcome shortcut around today's information overload, because it gives them the most important research from dozens of leading experts woven together with its own empowering perspectives on bringing more joy into family life. http://marcyaxness.com/book/

So what can you do to nurture that bond with your newborn? Find a way to take advantage of the hormonal cocktail that puts you in the right frame of mind and body to fall in love with your baby. Simplify your life so that the everyday ups and downs do not interfere with the connection you are fostering. Maybe a postpartum doula is the answer, since she can take care of the housework and other children allowing you and your baby to get to know each other. Resist the temptation to be on the phone, Facebook, Twitter, or the internet while you are breastfeeding or interacting with your baby. Being present with your baby is essential. Try the energy medicine techniques in the next chapter.

The time you invest in these early days will bring great dividends down the road when you have a secure child who is able to embrace the world with confidence and curiosity. This is the generation that will cultivate peace for the world based on their upbringing of loving connection with their parents. I resonate with Axness about elevating humanity through the mother and child communion. One last quote from her excellent book about what neuroscience is confirming are the ingredients for a healthy and happy human being: "relationship with a consistent, stable, attuned, loving adult, within a predictable, stable environment, is what builds a healthy brain and develops a successful human, period" (Axness, 2012, p. 397). Let this be your incentive for establishing and maintaining a loving and sensitive bond that becomes a lifelong positive attachment to your child and a model for future relationships.

CHAPTER 22

Energy Medicine for Bonding and Attachment – Radiant Circuits

One of the nine systems of Eden Energy Medicine is called Radiant Circuits, and they work like website hyperlinks, jumping wherever the body needs their joyful energy and revitalization. Unlike meridians that have fixed energy pathways, radiant circuits are like a reservoir of energy that lies dormant until they are required. They have a spontaneous intelligence that links up all the energy systems using the principle of harmony. From an evolutionary perspective, radiant circuits have been around longer than meridians and can be seen in primitive organisms that don't have meridians. They are called circuits because they can create instant circuits for the redistribution of energy to wherever they are most needed in the body. They carry a radiant glow as they make their connections, and they can channel healing energies into the body, and reorient the psyche for joy over despair. Not only do they do repair work, but they are also the primary energies of exhilaration, orgasm, hope, rapture, spiritual ecstasy, and gratitude.

Sometimes referred to as psychic circuits, they are instantly responsive to what you think and are associated with the awakening of psychic abilities. This is an obvious enhancement for your maternal instincts and intuition. Radiant circuits are the energetic bridge between what you think and the activation of neurotransmitters in the brain, and they can repattern brain pathways for joy at your neurological foundations.

Radiant circuits are an excellent energy-medicine technique for bonding and attachment because "the radiant circuits mobilize your *inner mom,* showering you with healing energy, providing life-sustaining resources, and lifting your morale" (emphasis mine; Eden & Feinstein, 2009, pp. 32-33). What could be better than to share that radiant energy with your newborn and with your partner as you are forming lifelong bonds?

Your radiant energy can also activate radiance in the baby. During fetal development, radiant circuits are the first energy circuit to appear in the embryo, before meridians. Babies see, feel, sense, and know energy when they are born, and they see the energies that surround you. This is why it always seems as if they are looking at the edges of your head and body. Activating radiant circuits can help to shift your deep habits and persistent negative thinking with their spontaneous, joyful waves of healing energy, leading to inner peace and greater enjoyment of life. They attract uplifting circumstances and events, in addition to connecting the energies in the body. I believe this could be a great starting point for women who have experienced a traumatic birth experience, though it might have limitations in dealing with the more distressing features of posttraumatic stress disorder (PTSD).

Techniques

The **9 Hearts Exercise** that we did in Part 3 is one way of activating your radiant circuits. Some of the exercises from the Daily Energy Routine (go to Chapter 5 for the instructions) are great ways of jumpstarting (never was a term more accurate in describing the way this energy moves) the radiant circuits. The **Hook Up** is one of them, and it connects your yin and yang energies, held for one to two minutes, after doing the **4 Thumps** and a **Zip-Up**. **Connecting Heaven and Earth** activates the spleen as a radiant circuit. **Heaven Rushing In** is another and helps to open your mind to the bigger picture.

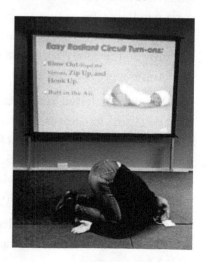

There is another easy turn-on of radiant circuits called **Butt in the Air**. The picture of me shows the position, although you will start off with your butt resting on your heels. This position transforms stress into a sense of security and safety. Starting on all fours, push back until your butt rests on your heels, bring your hands to your sides, and gently lower your head to the floor/ground. If you are comfortable doing it, move your body and head forward to lay your face to one side so your butt can go higher (this is the position I'm in). Hold this for 2 to 3 minutes. You can use this time to think about something positive and joyful, or just let your mind wander.

Another great movement to do for turning on radiant circuits is **Dancing to the Eights (8s).** The body's aura is composed of energy that moves in figure-8 shapes, which is one of nature's most basic patterns and can be found in the DNA double helix. When you consciously weave your energies in figure-8 curves, it brings greater health and vitality to the body as it activates the radiant circuits. Find some music that will energize you and start moving your hips in figure-8 patterns from side to side, and front to back. Be creative with this and then start using your arms, drawing figure-8s in the air in front of you, and then all around. Let your whole body move and experiment with large ones and small ones, whatever feels right to you. Have fun and be radiant.

Several radiant circuits connect front and back, and top to bottom, and the one that we will focus on now is called **Penetrating Flow**, which directs energy more deeply inward. It penetrates the chakras, muscles, bones, genitals, and down into the cells when it is moving freely. When it is blocked or weak, people can feel depressed, so it's good to activate penetrating flow because it can convey a deep sense of purpose and meaning to life. The 9 Hearts exercise also gets penetrating flow going. To activate penetrating flow, this exercise starts with you lying on your back with your legs bent at the knees and with your feet crossed at the ankles. Grasp your left foot with your right hand, and your right foot with your left hand (crossing over is always good for energy flow). Pull your feet up towards your head and keep the arms straight, and rock on your back so the butt comes off the ground. Continue rocking as long as you want and then rest in this position. There is a point on the back, directly behind your navel, called **Mingmen**, which is the source of the penetrating flow (image 18 shows the point from the back, image 19 from the side on the next page). When you rock in this way, you are stimulating Mingmen and the flow of energy through this circuit.

PART 5 INTRODUCTION

When I first started writing and teaching about a couple's relationship approaching the birth of their first child, there were few resources for this topic. It became a strong focus in The Birth Empowerment Workshop˚, which was born in 1988. This has changed over the last 30 years with a great influx of information available not only about relationships in general but also about the profound impact of birth on the relationship of new parents, with statistics to go with them. We will explore those aspects and develop strategies for keeping you connected while you expand your family, recognizing that the postpartum period is the most challenging time for everyone.

Amid all the adjustments, I can't stress enough how important it is to set time aside every week for your relationship. Even if it's just holding hands while you watch television together in the early weeks, this regular reconnection will keep your relationship humming through the turbulence. Finding ways to work as a team will increase your appreciation of each other at a time when it is so easy to draw the wrong conclusions about the other's experience and motives.

The truth is that couples' relationships break down all too often in the early years after a baby is born. The dramatic changes that happen to us as individuals, and as couples, can drive a wedge between us. So many things contribute to relationship stress after birth. The birth itself and the level of support that was felt. The kind of family we come from and our upbringing and belief system. How we were parented and issues from our early childhood that are recreated when our child is born. And how these individual backgrounds blend in the couple's relationship once they become parents. Relationship functioning also plays a role in perinatal mental illness because adult attachment can support or undermine the early co-parenting experience.

However, the transition to parenthood is ripe for more secure partner bonding: bonding with each other as we bond to our babies. This Part of the book provides creative strategies as an antidote to relationship stress. Take advantage of this window of opportunity to strengthen the partner relationship while welcoming a new person into the family. We'll start with communication because it is the bedrock on which intimacy is based.

CHAPTER 23

Communication

The Elements of Open Communication

Communication is the process by which we send and receive messages, and how we make contact with others. In the process of communicating, we exchange signals, sometimes verbally and always nonverbally. Even when we aren't conscious of the body language we transmit, so much between people is left unsaid. Communication implies that more than one person is involved: one who is expressing, and the other who is responding or listening, when it's a one-to-one exchange.

Communication also happens in groups or as one person to many, when there is an audience, such as during a lecture or workshop. In any case, we are attempting to make explicit whatever our thoughts and expectations are, though sometimes we are more effective than others. Often, there is the presumption that the other person will be able to read our minds and know how we are feeling or what we want, that our feelings or expectations are obvious, and they can figure it out. However, communication does not work based on supposition, and we are *not* mind-readers. We are ordinary humans. Our assumptions are unfounded (more often than not) and I am reminded of a useful slogan I learned when I was quite young: when you assume, you make an ass out of you and me (ass/u/me). That statement has served me well over the years and has helped me to not make assumptions most of the time.

To truly communicate, there must be at least two people fully engaged in the exchange, and we need to step up to the interaction. Often, our conditioning teaches us to keep our mouths shut and hide our true feelings. Perhaps we were scolded as children for being rude when we spoke out. The reinforcement for not saying anything unless it's nice (if you can't

and pleasurable feelings. No wonder so many of us are uncomfortable expressing affection. I know since the vast majority of my generation were not breastfed, we missed out on the opportunity to experience close intimate body contact as infants, where the warmth of skin touching is understood deep in our body consciousness as divine pleasure.

As already described in earlier chapters, nursing is how we develop the ability to be in close physical contact with others. Breastfeeding is the first language we understand, of skin to skin, where intimacy is known before words can create distance. It is an opportunity to be brought together and know the unity of nurturing that nursing reinforces. We need to awaken our senses and receive pleasure once again because when there is a sensuous exchange between partners, we manifest our physical expression of caring.

The Five Principles of Effective Communication

The following principles of effective communication are adapted from the book *Open Marriage*, by Nena and George O'Neill (1972). There was a lot of misunderstanding about what the purpose of *Open Marriage* was, and it developed a reputation of being about open, sexual freedom within marriage (which isn't even mentioned until the last eleven pages of the book). In fact, the book was one of the first to present options for open communication and an open relationship based on equal freedom and identity for both partners. You can use these guidelines during that inevitable time after the baby arrives, when both of you are being stretched to expand your identities within the stressful context of newborn parenting. Be fair, and you'll transcend these difficulties and reach a greater appreciation of each other as parents, with less need to criticize and judge each other's actions or motives.

The five principles of effective communication are essential factors in the art of communication. They are:

1. **Understand the context:** This means that we interact within a web of circumstances that bring meaning to our experience. We need to be sensitive to these conditions in what we say, as it will

increase our awareness of the perspective of the other person, as well as the background that shapes the issue.

2. **Timing:** It's important to choose the timing of this communication to be the best moment for both of us to fully and openly discuss our concerns. By attuning to our partner's moods and nonverbal gestures, we can choose a time that will further honest communication. Be sure not to use timing in a negative, manipulative way. Tipping the scales in our favor and catching our partner off guard is not being respectful of proper timing.

3. **Clarity:** Being very clear on what we have to say ensures that each of us will fully understand what's up for discussion. The tendency to be accusatory in our approach only makes the other person feel attacked. If, on the other hand, we merely express how we feel, the other person can hear the words without emotionally shutting down.

"Say what you see, tell what you feel, but do not criticize" are the famous words of Dr. Haim Ginott, who wrote extensively on communication in his many books, most notably *Between Parent and Child* (1965). Ginott felt communication flows best in an atmosphere of "emotional hospitality," which allows for telling it like it is, without criticism or judgment. By describing the situation, we can communicate what needs to happen without telling someone what to do, which most people hate. I was fortunate to have taken workshops with one of his disciples, Elaine Mazlish, when I was pregnant with my second child. Elaine and her co-author Adele Faber have written several books themselves on parent/child communication.

4. **Open listening:** This principle expands upon what we've already discussed on listening. It is sometimes referred to as active listening, and when we are doing it, we are more able to hear. When we are in genuine dialogue with another, we both listen and respond to one another with complete openness, and this kind of listening moves the conversation beyond communication to communion. Communion brings us closer to unity, and it expands to a feeling of connection to all of humanity on a spiritual level.

5. **Feedback:** Any open communication will include feedback, indicating that the other person understands what has been said, tells us how the other person feels, and makes it possible for us to adjust our feelings and perceptions on a realistic basis. Feedback can be given in the following forms: by paraphrasing, asking questions of clarification, or making a responsive statement saying how we feel. Feedback is how we gain closure around our interaction.

The five principles allow us to continuously grow in our ability to communicate, with a clean, healthy approach to working on our personal growing edge (the place of vulnerability where we take risks to develop) in a climate of acceptance and sharing. Feelings can be withheld in communication because we assume (there's that word again) that they have conflict-producing potential. By disclosing our feelings, we can invite clarification in a sharing context. During The Birth Empowerment Workshop`, we do an exercise called "sharing withholds" to do just that. It cleans up any unfinished business in the relationship and allows couples to really listen without getting defensive because when one person shares, the other person just says "thank you," and nothing more. After three rounds of each sharing one thing, they can then elaborate and clarify on the things they've shared. It really is effective.

Developing Synergy – The "We" System

Who we are, and how we relate, is determined by the historical, social, and natural forces acting on and within us. This includes the cultural impact, family history, and inner drives that define the roles we take on. Men who believe that sensitivity is a form of weakness become inducted into a macho stereotype of masculinity. The power of the feminine has been diminished in most patriarchal cultures, and this often contributes to rigid roles between the sexes (previously called sex-role stereotypes, they are now gender roles). Some women need to allow their strong, assertive nature to surface, and some men need to be tender and responsive. These contrasexual aspects of ourselves urge us into new ways of being and new forms of communication as integrated wholes. Our ability to communicate within our relationships provides us with a bridge that connects one state of our being with a new awareness as we become parents. The smoothness of the transition depends on the quality of the relationship and the clarity of the communication.

Synergy is a dynamic process in which two individuals (or things) come together so that the whole becomes more than the sum of its parts, while the individuals retain their own individuality: "that one plus one equals more than two, that the sum of the parts working together is greater than the sum of the parts working separately" (O'Neill & O'Neill, 1972, p. 39). Synergy is another term for the "we system," or the combined energy of two people working together to create an honest relationship of unity based on personal intimacy.

There are many different styles of relating, and with nonverbal communication representing about 70% of all communication, it speaks our truth, even when words are inadequate to express how we feel, or we feel unable to voice them. Therefore, it's essential to begin to learn how to read the energy that is being expressed through nonverbal communication. We must do that when our babies are born (check out The Blossom Method in Chapter 19) and we can extend that to include becoming more attuned to what we are picking up in the way of unspoken needs, desires, or feelings in our partners (the energy-medicine techniques at the end of this chapter will help with that too).

Working together as a team is better than working separately during the demands of the newborn period, which will go a long way to preventing the common resentments felt by one person feeling they are doing all the work during this intense time. One great way to establish synergy is through cyclical breathing with our partners. It means spending a few minutes together doing synchronized breathing, pacing each other, and breathing in slowly and breathing out slowly. You can place your hand on your partner's chest to help pace the rhythm, and soon, you will feel that team energy returning between you.

Divergent Styles of Communicating

Over the years, certain stereotypes have emerged along the lines of "men are from Mars and women are from Venus." I haven't read John Gray's books, but I have read Deborah Tannen, who wrote the classic book *You Just Don't Understand* (1990), which explores gender differences in communication

CHAPTER 24

Conscious Loving, Commitment, and Friendship

As co-leaders in the relationship field, Gay and Katie Hendricks, with their book *Conscious Loving: The Journey to Co-Commitment* (1990), created a system for transforming unconscious loving, with all the powerful influences from the past that are embedded in the way we connect with others, into conscious co-commitment. As they explain in their classic book, to commit is to bring together, and making a commitment is the essential task in resolving any conflict or problem that might be interfering with being a conscious partner. They also describe that there are specific requirements to making these commitments: we need to feel all our feelings, tell the microscopic truth (speaking the truth about our inner experience as we perceive it, without judgment or interpretation), and keep our agreements. These are the essential ingredients for commitment as they see it.

Co-commitments are "I" statements, the way for us to take responsibility for our actions and attitudes. We cannot project our undesirable parts on to our partner when we are coming from this place of what I will do, say, or be. As we each take ownership of our desires, we open the space to harmonize our goals and expectations from a place of wholeness. By focusing on our own part in the issue, we can get to the heart of the matter without making assumptions or attributing incorrect motives to our partner. With each person inquiring within, we can then bring our answers to a conversation in which we reveal a more accurate picture of the situation from our own perspectives.

Your partner can do the same, and this will definitely uplift the conversation to one where solutions are co-created, and a third way is found; not yours or your partner's, but a combined outlook that incorporates the truth for both of you. It shifts the consciousness from an either/or perspective to a both/and viewpoint. This is a win-win situation for all, especially your new baby, who now has peaceful and reunited parents to learn about love from.

Because the newborn parenting experience is so fraught with tension, mainly from lack of sleep and inexperience, it is so easy to blame the other person as not meeting our expectations of how they should be doing things. "Should" is a trap we all fall into from time to time, and it expresses the unspoken rules we learned from other influential people in our lives. As a therapist, I have often provided an echo to my clients whose speech is peppered with shoulds. If I ask them to remove the shoulds from their vocabulary, they have real trouble getting their message across and find themselves stumbling over what words to say. However, it's a real eye-opener, and it helps them to see how they are living their lives according to someone else's dictates.

We don't realize how deeply embedded this programming is. Again, when dealing with shoulds, there is the issue of projection: externalizing what we absorbed in life onto others. "Dropping projection is perhaps the single most powerful action you can take to transform your relationship," said Gay and Katie Hendricks. By taking this course of action, you will also reduce the number of shoulds you place upon yourself and your partner. Their excellent book has a whole section on exercises you can do to increase the closeness between you and raise the relationship to a heightened level of awareness and a more profound commitment to each other. I highly recommend this book.

Friendship and the Four Horsemen of the Apocalypse

At the end of the 20th century, another leader in the relationship arena came to prominence: John Gottman, emeritus professor of psychology. He claims he can predict (with a 91% success rate) which marriages would fail or succeed based on the behaviors of each person. He could come to this conclusion after watching and listening to a couple for just five minutes in his "Love Lab" in Seattle, Washington. In his book, *The Seven Principles for Making Marriage Work* (1999), he dispels some myths about relationships, particularly with regard to conflict resolution: "successful conflict resolution isn't what makes marriages succeed" (Gottman & Silver, 1999, p. 11). In his research, he has found that when couples are upset, they rarely engage in active listening. This is something to bear in mind when you are feeling touchy and sensitive from lack of sleep or the constant demands of a newborn. He does acknowledge that people have different styles of conflict, but he would dispute the different-planets theory.

> The determining factor in whether wives feel satisfied with the sex, romance, and passion in their marriage is, by 70 percent, the quality of the couple's friendship. For men, the determining factor is, by 70 percent, the quality of the couple's friendship. So men and women come from the same planet after all (Gottman & Silver, 1999, p.17).

For Gottman, the vital element of a happy marriage is friendship, which he defines as mutual respect, the enjoyment of each other's company, knowing each other intimately concerning likes, dislikes, personality quirks, and hopes and dreams. Friendship protects us from feeling adversarial towards our partners and allows us to give each other the benefit of the doubt. Gottman calls this the "positive-sentiment override," and it means we can put a positive spin on our thoughts about each other and the relationship that outweighs any negative feelings.

Equally, there is also a "negative-sentiment override" that has the opposite effect, where everything is interpreted through a negative lens. By reinvigorating friendship in the relationship, and the positive regard that goes with it, the level of fighting is kept from getting out of control.

Other studies began to validate his results by the 1980s, and the crisis view of the transition to parenthood took hold. Gottman has corroborated this through numerous long-term studies of his own. In these studies, they found that parents fell into two categories: the "masters" who navigated their way through the transition with a certain degree of aplomb, and the "disasters" who became very unhappy with each other during this transitional time (and the latter were twice as many). The masters coped far better with the trials and tribulations of early parenthood, and much was learned from the masters.

And Baby Makes Three is the practical application of *The 7 Principles* within the context of new parenthood. Much of the material is repeated, so if you could only purchase one book, then *And Baby Makes Three* will also provide the content for working on the relationship. In their chapter on delighting in your baby, much of what is covered in this book is also presented there along with information about babies and their developmental needs. The new edition also incorporates new neuroscientific and physiological content that explains the biochemical experience that accompanies the management of conflict. They present what to do in the aftermath of a fight and how to process it, as well as the dangers of gridlock: "We pay a high price for gridlock. We end up feeling that our partner doesn't even like us, let alone love us. After a while, all our discussions lack humor, affection, curiosity, empathy, and even basic understanding" (Gottman & Gottman, 2007, p. 129).

Intimacy

A critical section of the Gottmans' book is their exploration of couples' intimacy experiences and the effect that having a baby has on your sex life. It isn't always recognized how breastfeeding can impact on your libido (desire for sex), or what the *lack* of hormones can do (e.g., when estrogen is low, this has a thinning effect on vaginal tissues). In their research, they found some interesting patterns between men and women three years after the baby was born. Three years later, women only felt a fraction of what their husbands felt regarding frequency in the desire for sex, and the same pattern was evident in how much sexual touch they wanted.

When rating themselves on how sexual they felt, women felt "not very," and men rated themselves as "extremely" sexual. The theory that developed from many studies of couples is: "Many couples sexually disconnect after Baby is born, and that gap may last for as long as three years! Before Baby, most everybody wants sex. After Baby, men want sex a lot more than women" (Gottman & Gottman, 2007, p. 160). I'm glad to see the evidence that proves what I have observed for nearly 40 years with my clients. The authors acknowledge the biological influence but also indicate that sexual feelings reflect relationship satisfaction, and when closeness decreases, sexual desire dries up too (pun intended). And before you jump down my throat because this doesn't apply to you, there are some couples where the situation is reversed, and women want sex more than their husbands, and there are also couples whose sex life flowered when they became a family.

The master couples were able to bring their sexual intimacy back to life through nonsexual affectionate touching, with no expectation that it would lead to something more sexual. Women cherish receiving affection, but it is often a matter of confusion for men, who conflate intimacy with sex. The Gottmans found that all positive interactions, especially appreciations, are foreplay. There are gender differences in play—she's a Dutch oven, for whom sex is a slow buildup, and he's a microwave, and sex is a quick release. I love these analogies, so apt not just after the baby, but in life, generally.

Touch

Tenderness is the expression of warm affection in our relationships, and a highly effective way of opening or maintaining open communication. It provides the environment in which we can be uninhibited in how we express ourselves, opening the space for feelings, fears, desires, and expectations to be revealed and corroborated. Remember, we cannot work based on supposition, and mindreading is not an ordinary human capacity. Tenderness also works wonders for attracting physical intimacy because it brings us into an expanded awareness of touch: how we like to be touched and how we perceive our partners want to be touched. In touching each other, we learn how each of us defines different qualities of touch, and we gain confidence in knowing how to please the other.

Through touch, we know that we are allies and not adversaries. Touch is our most intimate form of communication, and our ability to be sensuous in a relationship depends on our tactile sense being stimulated. However, there is one caveat here. Through breastfeeding, many postpartum women can feel touched out in the early days and are likely to be less receptive to touch with their partners. Forty-five years ago, the O'Neills wrote: "Couples need to relearn the full use of physical expression as a means of intimate communication and to reawaken their sensuality" (O'Neill & O'Neill, 1972, p. 103). Because for so many of us, the deep need for physical intimacy has been conditioned out of us, and we need to reawaken our physical senses and the touch receptors that were desensitized by cultural disapproval during our childhood conditioning. Society has a strong influence on our ability to receive pleasure, and this has been going on since the Victorian days. Sam Keen, a wonderful author who I've mentioned earlier, philosopher, and once editor of *Psychology Today* for 20 years, spoke very specifically to this matter in his excellent book, *The Passionate Life: Stages of Loving* (1983):

> In the measure that our myth has valued masculine achievement over feminine being, it has woven a punishing set of rationalizations into its views about birth, childcare, touch, and sensuality. A generation ago, my mother heeded the best medical advice and listened in agony while I cried and waited to feed me until the schedule said I should eat. Nudity and fondling within the family were forbidden by Puritans and orthodox Freudians because they supposedly invited incest. Generation after generation we produce children who are poorly bonded because their parents were terrified of their own sensuality. Gradually, the body politic increases its disposition toward obsessive sexuality (the compensation for the dearth of touch) and violence (Keen, 1983, p. 55).

Over 35 years later, this quote still has resonance. I had the privilege of taking part in a workshop with Sam Keen when my son Jasper was about 6 months old, and I remember having to go into the bathroom to pump my milk because I was breastfeeding. In fact, that was one of the only times that I did pump (it wasn't very effective) because I found manual expression to be very efficient, but since I was away from my baby for a full day, I thought I'd try pumping. Sam called me a "passionate pilgrim," and he is an inspiration with a gifted mind.

We need to become lovers again, so that our children can inherit a sensuous legacy from us, to take delight in the pleasure of tender touch, and to know the joy of comfort received in loving arms. Then, our children can mature into lovers who know the joy of lovemaking instead of gratuitous sex, and while appreciating the value of touch, can then encounter intimacy with less withholding and more openhearted love. The level of intimacy we can share with each other will impact strongly on how loving we can be with our children. By bringing open hearts into our relationships, we express the deepest levels of intimacy (into-me-see) with those we love, and that will always be easier with loved ones who are able to accept us as whole individuals. When we model positive communication skills to those with whom we interact, it becomes contagious.

Sex

Another area where the Gottmans and I agree is in finding alternative ways of expressing sexual fulfillment outside of sexual intercourse. I don't know why penetration is viewed as the gold standard of pleasure for couples, in an all-or-nothing way, because there are so many ways that we can pleasure each other to keep the juices flowing when intercourse is not recommended in the early postpartum period. We can honor our partner's wishes and needs, and keep the embers alive until the time is right to resume sexual intercourse. And for a while after that happens, sex might be more like a quickie (Why do babies seem to have radar about when parents are getting in the mood? Is it the oxytocin they can smell?), rather than the delicious, languid sex that we can enjoy when we are not likely to be interrupted. It can be great fun to explore other forms of pleasure in our primary relationship, and this is more likely if affection has been shared and tenderness cultivated (between parents, as well as towards the baby).

Maintaining contact keeps us connected with each other, and acts as the pilot light for when sexual arousal is ignited. Make a game out of finding out various interesting ways of giving pleasure to each other. In Chapter 22, I talked about the Mingmen point, at the middle of the lower back directly behind the navel and how to activate it, in the energy-medicine section on radiant circuits. It is part of Traditional Chinese Medicine (TCM) and is called The Gate of Life, and it holds the energies of yin and yang in harmony. It is the source of penetrating flow, acting like a switching station that sends energy to the organs and supports rejuvenation and revitalization.

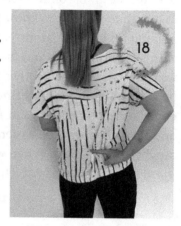

As I explained in the chapter, penetrating flow is one of the radiant circuits of the body, the "inner wells of joy" that infuse strength, resilience, spontaneous healing, and vitality into the body. Long before I knew about Mingmen, I was aware that this part of my body was very sensitive to gentle touch. Why don't you see how your body responds to touch in this area as gentle as a feather? You might be very pleasantly surprised at your response.

Some of the issues of newborn parenting, which we have covered in other chapters, include: sleep deprivation that makes every little thing seem exaggerated, the division of labor that shifts after a baby is born and needs to be renegotiated, changes in relationship needs (often downward), such as sex, sharing, and appreciation, which ups the ante on conflicts, and the desire to be good parents to our babies so they can thrive. It's like moving through a maelstrom at times, and it's hard to find our center when we are whirling dervishes through the labyrinth of new parenting during the postpartum period. At times, it becomes hard to remember who the baby is and who the parents are, as everyone is needy. For our children to grow up healthy, strong, and emotionally intelligent, they need us to maintain loving and healthy relationships with each other. Life is challenging, but in much the same way that the Chinese kanji (symbol) for crisis has two parts: danger and opportunity, your new life with a baby is multifaceted. There are challenges, stresses, powerful emotions, hard work, and hassles, and there are joys and fulfillment too. When we operate as a duet and share the load, the transition becomes so much more manageable. We nurture our relationship so we can nourish our baby.

Why Dads Leave

The quote from Sam Keen above, describing how children were poorly bonded in generations past due to restricted ideas about how much sensuality was permitted, raises an important issue that is not well-known or understood about fathers and partners. Nearly 30 years later, Meryn G. Callander and contributor John W. Travis wrote a detailed account of the Dynamic of Disappearing Dads (DDD), which John labeled Male Postpartum Abandonment Syndrome (MPAS) in their book *Why Dads Leave* (2012). I had the good fortune to meet Jack at his workshop on these phenomena at the BirthKeeper Summit in 2015, and we've been communicating ever since. A leader in the wellness movement going back to the 1970s, he opened the first wellness center in 1975 (Mill Valley, California). Jack was astounded to find new parenthood so psychologically challenging.

With his second child (born to Meryn, 21 years after his first daughter), they had the expectation of a very different outcome due to their understanding of how an insecure mother/infant bond is the most significant impediment to wellbeing. Instead, Jack began withdrawing from his wife emotionally, along with bouts of depression, recapitulating the experience he encountered after his first child was born. This led him to explore more deeply what was going on with himself. He was aware that when the father has a history of unmet needs from his own infancy and childhood, these are often activated with the birth of his own child, as the baby is now receiving all the nurturing that he had depended on before. This re-stimulation of childhood wounding stirs an often-unconscious awareness of what he didn't get, and he often copes by leaving emotionally, or even physically.

His self-exploration started out as a newsletter article called "Why Men Leave: Confessions of a Bottle-Fed, Circumcised, Poorly Bonded, Depressed, Thrice-Married, White Male Semi-Reformed Overachiever" (1998) and was expanded for publication in parenting magazines in the U.S. and Australia in 2004. It became the premise of their book, *Why Dads Leave* after one of the magazine editors reported that the article had generated the strongest reader response ever. Apparently, they had touched a nerve for other men who had similar experiences.

The book is a compendium of research and personal stories about the developmental and attachment needs of all humans. It synthesizes theories and models from a wide range of sources on pregnancy, birth, parenting, relationships, and healing. What is unique to this book is the definition and examination of the Male Postpartum Abandonment Syndrome (MPAS) that causes the epidemic of disappearing marriages. It explains a great deal about the lingering impact on fathers who were not securely bonded to their caregivers in early life. While mothers may be healing their own wounds of disconnection through the closer physical bond they experience with their children, from carrying and then nursing them, the fathers' reaction to the birth of his child can have profound unconscious origins that manifest in an assortment of behaviors that create distance within the couple.

Why Dads Leave explores "the factors that arise and may lead to a couple separating in the early years after the birth of a child" (Callander, 2012, p. 25), and how MPAS exposes how the cultural mass disconnection and failure to bond is self-perpetuating. As we saw in Part 4, bonding and attachment are crucial processes that connect families, and understanding some of the lifelong patterns that can interfere with these developments allows us to stay compassionately engaged enough to express feelings of rejection, abandonment, and loss.

The Adult Attachment bond can be transformed within the couple relationship so that everyone's needs are being met. The book includes numerous strategies for healing, such as inner child work, exercises to work with relationship reactivity, and dialogues with internal guidance systems. It also reveals some of the shame that men experience in their relationships with women and ways to reduce the shame and develop a friendship between partners, something that Gottman espoused above.

CHAPTER 25

Becoming Us™ as Parents

In 2012, I had the honor to meet and work with Elly Taylor, relationship counselor and author of *Becoming Us: 8 Steps to Grow a Family that Thrives* (2014). As is often the case these days, we met online in a Facebook group. We were coming from the same page in focusing our attention on the relationship issues of couples becoming parents. She wrote a book about it, and I created a couple's retreat called The Birth Empowerment Workshop*. We created our own group on Facebook called Relationship-Focused Birth Professionals and collaborated on a workshop presented at the 2013 18th International Congress of the Association for Prenatal and Perinatal Psychology and Health. The workshop called "Fostering the Couple Connection in the Transition to Parenthood" combined our individual expertise for helping other professionals to empower childbearing families. This was followed by a poster session we created for the International Marcé Society for Perinatal Mental Health conference in 2014, "Strengthening the Adult Attachment Bond to Reduce the Risk of Perinatal Mood Disorders for Mothers & Fathers/Partners."

Elly's is a wonderful book on "loving, learning, and growing together" as parents. I think it should be required reading for new parents because it covers so much of the territory of how relationships transform during this important transition, and it offers lots of strategies for dealing with the common issues of adjusting to parenthood. Inspired by her own experience of realizing "I don't know how to do this," I think she speaks for the vast majority of new parents whose lives are thrown into a tailspin by the arrival of a baby. Her motivation for writing her book is like the motivation I had for writing this book on the postpartum experience: "somebody should write a book about this stuff."

of the normal challenges that couples experience as they move through the stages of a relationship and how they can work through them. Also, it provides a framework for empathetic counseling of couples during pregnancy in the form of pre-parenting preparation. So many of the crises of the transition to parenthood can be avoided when couples are prepared for what's to come and have the tools to work together as a duet. It has extended my understanding of attachment theory, particularly about the Adult Attachment bond between partners. When this partner bond is protected, and when we tend to it and help it grow, this connection becomes a strong foundation for the whole family.

One activity that is part of the Birth Empowerment Workshop° is a planting-seeds exercise with my couples, who were planting seeds for their family life together. The Becoming Us™ training also uses the metaphor of planting seeds for growth, and how to relate using primary and secondary emotions and intimate communication guidelines. A significant piece is adjusting expectations for parenthood that are grounded in reality, and understanding which expectations are helpful and unhelpful. I am drawn to the strengths-based work with couples that Becoming Us™ is, harnessing the strengths and abilities of the individuals and the couple. In fact, parenthood preparation can lead to better birth outcomes.

The eight steps to grow a family that thrives from the Becoming Us™ model include:

1. **Prepare for Your Baby**. During pregnancy, use the wonderful Nest Building Plan. This seven-page document details all the specifics of your wants and desires after birth, for the mother, father/partner, and both in ways that fortify the relationship. It includes what to plan for, managing the division of labor, organizing who are the resources for support, and an abundance of other ideas for life after the baby.

2. **Build Your Nest**. This is when you take all the preparation from your plan and implement it once the baby is born. Get support from others for everyday things. This is time for resting, nesting, and bonding as you adjust to postpartum life.

3. **Manage Expectations**. Managing expectations is a fundamental part of a smooth transition. I so often hear women say, "all I ever

wanted was to be a mom, and it wasn't what I expected." Learning which expectations are helpful and which are unhelpful is a way to stay realistic because those unhelpful expectations can lead to difficulties. This is like the Expectations section of the Postpartum WELLNESS Plan (PWP) from Chapter 4.

4. **Set Up Base Camp.** This is when you establish your new normal (also in the PWP). Your baby is settling in, and you can begin to see beyond the walls of your home and focus on your own needs too. During this time, it is helpful to create positive eating, exercise, and stress relief habits that will reinforce your ability to cope with what life hands you.

5. **Embrace Your Emotions**. Having a baby will engender a mix of emotions based on our personal history, our relationship, and our capacity to express them. People are surprised by the normal mix of positive and negative emotions that surface in this highly charged time, when we are naturally more internally sensitive as well. Being sensitive to our partner so we feel safe to share emotions will bring the relationship to a whole new level.

6. **Welcome Your Parent Self**. The adjustment that comes with your new roles draws on an increased understanding between partners based on respect, appreciation, and support for each other. "Supported partners make awesome parents," according to Elly Taylor and the co-parenting journey begins here.

7. **Grow Together Through Differences**. Sleep deprivation, added stresses, and steep learning curves are all normal, and you want to be able to get closer, not further apart. Remember that 92% of couples experience an increase in conflict in the first year after a baby is born. Such a high figure means conflict is common, but it doesn't mean there's something wrong with your relationship, and learning intimate communication skills helps to minimize and manage the battles that crop up.

8. **Connect and Reconnect**. Gottman found that 67% of couples experienced a decline in marital satisfaction in the first three years after a baby is born. The Becoming Us™ model offers various ways to increase happiness and stay connected, as the

foundation for a family that thrives. You are creating your "Us" now (like the "We" in the PWP), and your baby will thank you for tending the bond between you as you bond to your baby too.

Knowing these stages and changes are normal takes the pressure off couples, increasing the chances of a smooth transition. Teamwork opens the door for dialog so that couples can work together to express their needs and wants, helping each other love, learn, and grow as "Us."

I've worked with couples through my classes and workshops for decades, and I found Elly Taylor's program to be an excellent synthesis of evidence that brings couples closer together as they become parents. I'm so fortunate to be able to bring this approach to "parenting as an adventure" to my clients locally and from afar. Whether I'm planting seeds, being a parenthood "tour guide," or a village elder through counseling, this work with parents makes a real difference in parental relationships. I recommend that you seek out a Certified Becoming Us™ facilitator in your area to experience the joy in pre-baby preparation. We need to prepare for the relationship challenges in parenthood as well as birth, and the Becoming Us™ Parents Program provides a delightful, experiential course for Before Baby, and After Baby, that joyfully does just that!

CHAPTER 26

The Energies of Relationships

The 5 Rhythms Model

As part of the training I've done in Eden Energy Medicine, I have been exploring the way relationships play out on an energetic level. It is best described as adding a whole new dimension to how our energies affect each other in relationships. We each have our own energy template, and as a couple, the relationship energy can reflect how our energies affect each other. If our energy is scrambled, that will affect our partner, and if our partner's energies are out of balance, that will affect us. We can be energetically out of sorts, and we can help our partners get their energies back into balance. The key is to keep the energy flowing; it is the nature of energy to move. When it stops moving and stagnates, that's when we start to have problems that can include physical symptoms, emotional issues, or mental difficulties. The healing involves making space for energy to flow within us and between us.

To understand how this works, let me give you a bit of the background in Traditional Chinese Medicine (TCM) that is the essence of The Five Rhythms model. According to this tradition, one becomes two becomes five. The All of Life (1) is divided into the two principles that oppose and balance each other: yin and yang (2). The symbol for yin/yang is the Tai Chi, which is a whole circle divided into two parts, one of which is white, and the other is black. However, within each half is a small circle of the opposite principle, so there is a white circle within the black, and a black circle within the white. This represents how all yin has some yang, and all yang has some yin, and they are continuously creating and consuming

The key to using the Five Element Model with people is found in the ancient Chinese belief that, as part of the Universe, we contain all of the elements within our being, and the elements qualify how energy flows in and through us" (Matthews, 2008, p.7).

As mentioned above, we each have a natural affinity to one or two of the elements, and they will have a dominant effect in how our energy flows at the physical and emotional levels, as well as how energy flows between us and our surroundings. This affinity will shape our perspective on life and how we interact with the world, how we react to stress, and our relationships with others.

When we understand our primary (and secondary) element and those of our important loved ones and friends, it hints at why we behave the way we do and how to smooth the way to harmony and balance between us. Some elemental relationships will move through the flow cycle, and others will move through the control cycle in the model described above. The study of the Five Rhythms/Elements is complex and wide-ranging and I'm only going to present a quick synopsis of the elements so that you can begin to grasp how you and your partner might resonate with them. There is a whole part of the model that I am not including, and this has to do with how the 12 meridians are associated with the elements. Each element has two meridians, except for fire, which has four. Rather than complicate matters, we will just focus on the elements themselves and the typical characteristics of each. Starting with water, the first element, I will move around the flow cycle with the core of features that describes each of the elements and see if you can recognize the picture that emerges for each.

Flow Cycle

Water: Winter, new beginnings, search for the truth, little structure; *paradox:* yearns for connection with others yet wants solitude; positive emotion – hope; negative emotion/ stress response – fear/paranoia. *Archetype:* baby, philosopher. People who are waters are philosophical, creative, and full of ideas but can become negative and suspicious.

Wood: Spring, growth, and expansion, willing to try what hasn't been done, very structured in an organic way; *paradox:* goes in dozens of directions while feeling trapped and confined, loves to compete and hates to lose; positive emotion – assertiveness; negative emotion/ stress response – anger, frustration/rage. *Archetype:* warrior, pioneer. People who are woods are doers, good planners, and can actualize a lot, but watch out for their temper.

Fire: Summer, manifestation at its peak, fun-loving, enthusiastic, not very structured; *paradox:* yearns for intimacy yet needs alone time or will lose self; positive emotion – joy; negative emotion/stress response – panic/ hysteria. *Archetype:* wizard, unconditional lover. People who are fires are very outgoing, now-people, expressive, popular, and inspiring, but can be scattered and overcommit.

Earth: Transition times of solstices and equinoxes, brings balance to all, nurturing others and facilitating change, their structure is unique with slow movement and pondering; *paradox:* responds to need but can become dependent on being needed; positive emotion – compassion; negative emotion/stress response – worry, codependency. *Archetype:* earth mother, peacemaker. People who are earths are compassionate and caring, but need time to ponder the meaning of change, are not very good with boundaries, and can suffer for identifying too much with people they help. They are perpetually in the middle.

Metal: Autumn, things begin to die back, harvest, death and regeneration, rigid structure; *paradox:* craves distance and solitude yet needs meaningful relationships; positive emotion – awe and reverence; negative emotion/stress response – sadness/grief and emptiness, withdraws. *Archetype:* synthesizer, alchemist. People who are metals see the whole cycle and grasp the lessons it provides, but have trouble letting go, and are perceived as controlling and perfectionistic.

In a nutshell, this gives a broad idea of some of the themes and qualities of each element. Have a little fun with this and think about the important people in your life and how they may resonate with any particular element and do it for yourself. The relationships that appear on the clockwise flow cycle are part of the nurturing cycle, the way one element feeds the next: 1) water with wood, 2) wood with fire, 3) fire with earth, 4) earth with metal, and 5) metal with water.

When these elemental relationships are in balance, the relationship will feel very nourishing. When they are out of balance, the relationship will restrict the flow of energy for one or both parties, causing tension and conflict. In this case, each element will express their particular style of stress response: water will get fearful and hopeless; wood will get angry and frustrated; fire will get panicky and hysterical; earth will worry and find themselves in the middle; and metal will feel grief and be unable to let go. Sound familiar? Can you spot yourself? Your partner? When I was first learning the Five Rhythms model, I could see that my typical stress response was anger, and therefore, I was a wood. I didn't resonate with all of the wood qualities, but I have been a pioneer in my day and I like to get things done.

Control Cycle

The control cycle of relationships, also called the destructive cycle, creates a star in the way the straight flow of energy moves from one element to another. It is called the control cycle because when working with the meridians, it is possible to sedate and strengthen a meridian by holding certain points on it. The first set of points, from the flow cycle, moves the energy around, but the second set of points is called the control points because they stabilize the energy by stopping the flow.

When in balance, these relationships are supportive and freeing, but when out of balance these relationships will be overcontrolling and inhibiting. They are: 1) water with fire, 2) fire with metal, 3) metal with wood, 4) wood with earth, and 5) earth with water. Does your relationship fall into these patterns? When two people share the same element, it has its own challenges because there's no dynamic from different elements interacting and the cyclical movement of energy on the flow or control cycles is not there.

Energy Testing for the Dominant Rhythm/Element

The way to energy test the element goes like this. You begin with the tester saying the stress emotion for each rhythm out loud, and then energy testing immediately (using the General Indicator test; the person extends their arm at shoulder height on an angle forward, **#20**, and the tester applies pressure above the wrist for two seconds, creating a circuit with the other hand, **#21**, on the person's other shoulder). First, you need to test the arm being extended by doing a simple true/false test, such as "your name is ... (actual name)," followed by "your name is ... (false)," and see how the arm responds. It should hold with the correct name and go down with the false.

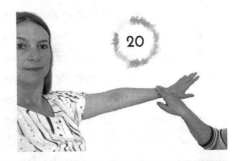

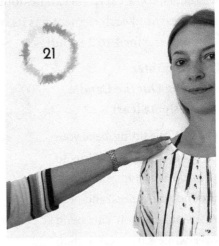

You can also turn the muscle off and on by pinching the muscle interior to the armpit, and then smoothing it out respectively. Once you have a reliable test, you can start to test the elements, being sure not to look the person in the eye, because it shifts the energy. Here's what you would say for each element: Water = **fear**; Wood = **anger**; Fire = **panic**; Earth = **worry**; Metal = **grief**. If the test shows weakness for an element, it could be dominant in the person's character or dominant in that moment in time. The stress emotion is a point of vulnerability for a rhythm, so a **weak test** (meaning the person is unable to hold the arm up and it goes down under pressure) on the stress emotion suggests that the rhythm is active. You can have some fun with each other testing for the different elements by using the stress response for each one.

Exercises for Balancing Elemental Energies

When there are relationship difficulties, it can signpost that an element is out of balance for one or both partners. When there are emotional and psychological issues, someone is having balance problems with an element. When there are inappropriate behaviors or strong emotional reactions to things, this is an indication that one or more elements are out of balance. By observing, you can make some common connotations about yourself and your partner. When you want to change the energy balance in specific elements, some exercises can be done to balance the energies and reduce the stress, and each element has its own exercise. Each of these exercises can be done for **1 to 2 minutes**.

Water/Winter –
Blowing Out the Candle
(to dissipate fear)

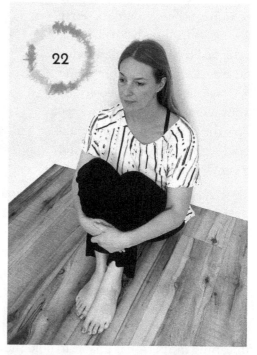

(#22) While sitting, bend your knees and raise your legs to your chest, wrap your arms around your knees, and hold. Alternatively, you can bend over while sitting on a chair and hold your arms around your bent knees. Take a deep breath and rock back and forth with your head lifted and staring at the imaginary blue flame of a candle. When you exhale throughout this exercise, let the air move through your puckered lips, making a soft whispered "Wooooo" sound of blowing out a candle. Continue to rock and blow until you no longer feel as fearful, as if the fear is going out with the flame.

Wood/Spring – *Expelling the Venom, also called Blow Out* (to dissipate anger)

Stand with feet parallel, about 1 to 2 feet apart, and hands on the thighs, fingers spread, take a deep breath. When you exhale, make a "Shhhhhhhhh" sound as if telling someone to be quiet. Position both arms bent in front of you (**#23**), with your hands in fists facing upwards. While inhaling deeply, swing the arms out to the sides and bring them high above your head. Recall the cause of the anger and make your movements quick and forceful.

Turn your hands so the wrists are facing each other (**#24**), then powerfully and with the loud "Shhhhhhhhh" sound as you exhale, bring your fisted hands down quickly, opening the hands as they reach your thighs (**#25**). Repeat two more times, but on the third time, bring the arms/hands down slowly and deliberately, feeling your muscles and power unfolding. To anchor the effect, zip up when done. You can feel the tension dissolving and the anger dissipating.

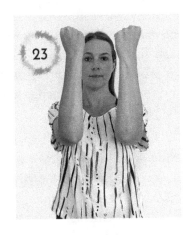

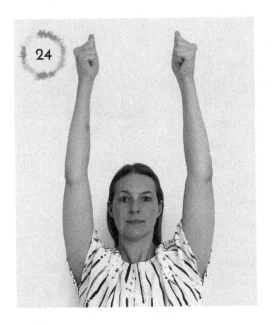

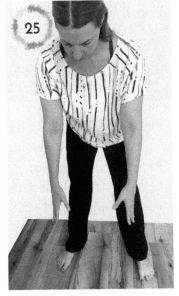

Fire/Summer – *Taking Down the Flame* (for panic or loss of spirit)

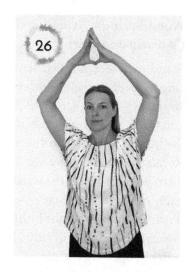

Starting in the same position as for Expelling the Venom, place your open hands on your thighs and sense the energy traveling down your legs and grounding you. Breathing deeply throughout this exercise, make a sighing "Haaaaaaa" sound with each exhale. Imagine the mental chaos or clutter dissolving with each sigh. Inhale deeply and circle the arms overhead, and bring the fingertips and thumbs of your hands together in a steeple (**#26**).

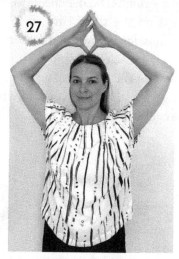

Exhaling with the "Haaaaaaa" sound, bring your thumbs down to the **crown chakra** at the center of the top of your head (**#27**), all fingers touching (throughout all the movements). Remain there and inhale. Exhaling with the "Haaaaaaa" sound, bring the thumbs to the **third eye** between your eyebrows (**#28**), and stay in this position as you inhale. Exhaling with the "Haaaaaaa" sound, bring your thumbs to the **heart chakra** between your breasts, and inhale as your stay there. Exhaling with the "Haaaaaaa" sound, bring the thumbs to the **navel**, and roll the hands down to form a pyramid (**#29**) beneath the navel. Maintain this position as you inhale, and with the next exhale and "Haaaaaaa" sound, flatten the hands[#30] and stretch them down to the original position on the thighs. Hold this position and inhale. Exhaling with the "Haaaaaaa"

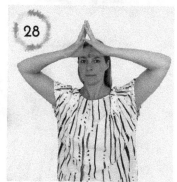

sound, slowly move your open hands down the legs as you bend over, and then let your hands hang down as you breathe in. Exhale with the sound while hanging over, and while inhaling, come up to a stand, bringing your hands up the inside of your legs to the original position. Exhale with the final sound.

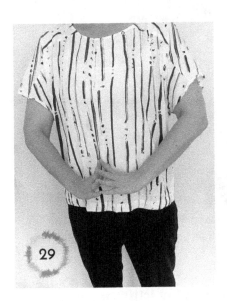

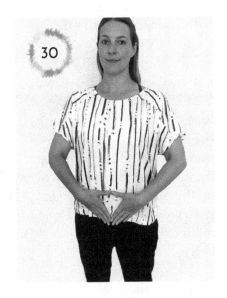

Earth/Solstice/Equinox – *Cradling the Baby* (for over-compassion)

Standing with your hands over your solar plexus, tenderly cradle your midsection as if it were a baby you are rocking (**#31**). You are bringing the sympathy you give to others back to yourself. Take a slow controlled breath in from the back of your throat, and exhale the same way from the back of the throat, making a raspy sound like "Eghhhh," and continue breathing in and out this way until you feel centered, and continue breathing this way with the movements. Inhale and circle your arms

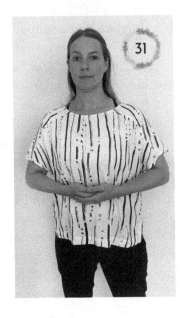

above your head and stretch one arm up and then the other up, twice for each side. Exhale and bend forward, reaching your arms forward and down, and placing the fingers of each hand underneath the inside arches of your feet (#32). Pull up while holding until you feel a stretch across your back and continue for a couple of raspy breaths. Then, inhale with the breathing and return to a stand while pulling hands up the insides of the legs, and then up the center of the body and

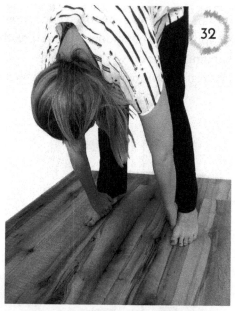

stretch overhead again. Exhale and return your hands to cradling your midsection at the solar plexus. Repeat until you can feel a shift in your energy.

Metal/Autumn – *Human Touching Divine* (for letting go and grief)

The trick to this exercise is inhaling with opening arms and exhaling with rounding arms. Stand straight and round your arms in front of you, bringing your fingers to almost touching each other (#33). Imagine you are holding the world and its problems. Inhale deeply and exhale, making a "Sssssss" sound, like air escaping a balloon. Inhale, opening your arms, releasing, surrendering, and letting go of the world, while you lift your chest and look up (#34).

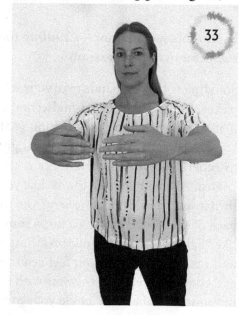

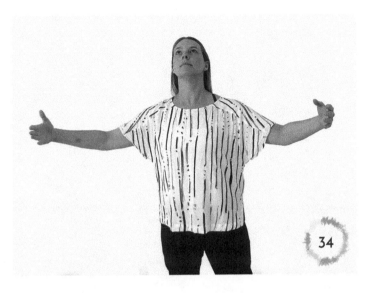

Exhaling with the "Sssssss" sound, round your arms in front and imagine the world you're holding, hands reaching but not touching. Inhale, open and release, and exhale but this time, the fingers touch (think of Michelangelo's fresco of God touching Adam) as they come together. Inhale and bring the world close to your chest (lungs hold grief) with your hands one on top of the other, holding tight to what you hold dear to you. With the last exhale and "Sssssss" sound, let it all go and open your arms out. You are letting go of the old and opening to the new. Repeat until there is a shift in the energy. With each out breath, draw to you what you love and have sorrow about. With each in breath, let it all go and open to belief and faith.

These activities are easy to do once you identify what the primary affinity is. However, just being able to understand how you or your partner's element is affecting the relationship gives you a basis for beginning to balance those energies. And if you haven't guessed what the essence of an energy-medicine approach to relationships is, it is balance.

Balancing the out of sync relationship, in this case by using the Five Rhythms/elements model, is the name of the game.

CHAPTER 27

Four Sensory Types

Eden Energy Medicine developed another energy-medicine approach to relationships that uses sensory types: visual, tonal, digital, and kinesthetic. These are based on the primary way that we process threat information through our senses, using our sensory systems, except for digital, which is about how we process information using thought. Our sensory systems allow us to receive input from the environment, which travels through neural pathways to the brain, where we interpret the data and create our perception of the world. We each have a sensory type that is dominant, and often, a secondary type that is powerful as well.

These sensory types can be thought of as representational systems, according to Neuro-Linguistic Programming (NLP), which is a model for how the human mind processes and stores information in sensorial terms from our experiences. The choice of words, phrases, and sentences used will generally give us a clue as to which representational system is operative or preferred. Visual types will use words that suggest images and vision. Tonals, or auditory (hearing) types, will use words that suggest sounds and hearing. Kinesthetic types will speak in terms of feelings and sensations. And digitals, who often are not feeling or tuned in to their senses, will use cognitive words expressing their rational point of view. Whichever system is preferred or dominant for us is the one that helps us to make sense of our experience, and has characteristic styles of interpretation called our Energetic Stress Style (Eden & Feinstein, 2014). In energy terms, it explains how our energies will be influenced by our sensory type.

Visuals: "I see"

Tonals: "I hear"

Kinesthetics: "I feel"

Digitals: "I think"

When we come into a relationship with someone, we are bringing two different energies together, and as the energies merge, they create a third energetic field out of the space between two people, which describes how it is experienced from moment to moment.

> The way your energy field and your partner's interact forms the framework for everything else about your relationship. It is the invisible force that supports your intimacy one moment but may place clouds of tension between you the next (Eden & Feinstein, 2014, p. 30).

This union of energies determines how we communicate, how we fight, and how we love and want to be loved. Relationships are about energy at a deeper level. The differences in our energies, our signature sensory styles, reflect how we each experience the world in different ways. They can indicate either irreconcilable differences or the spark that keeps a relationship interesting. We cannot make our partners think as we think, or want what we want, or perceive the way we perceive. The *Energies of Love* DVD by Eden and Feinstein (that preceded their more recent publication of *Energies of Love*, in 2014) shows how we can understand what happens when our sensory style meets another's sensory style and how to manage the energies of the two styles combined.

Energetically, we become a different person during relationship stress. When there is conflict or stress, if we can appreciate each other's energy style, we can anticipate how we are bound to respond or react, according to our sensory type. Each type will have specific features for meeting stress and a typical "modus operandi," so that being able to understand and work with the predominant style of our partners can enhance our compatibility.

It is also important to know that the characteristics of a sensory type extend beyond just the senses and involve our interpretations of the world. Because stress causes us to be thrown out of balance energetically, our perceptions can reflect how we are experiencing the world. In someone who is **visual**, energies in the body will concentrate in the head and upper chest during relationship stress, and move outward through the eyes, head, and chest. The **tonal** person has energy concentrating in two locations, 1) between and including the ears, and 2) the solar plexus, and this reverberates in the various organs in that area that controls strong emotions. The partner's comments can activate a rush of emotions that aren't even related to the words or intended meaning.

A **digital** under stress will have energy accumulating in the forebrain, and the body is cut off from the mind. The feelings of the digital's partner become irrelevant. The **kinesthetic** person has energies moving inward, and this includes the partner's energies, which are soaked up like a sponge. Energy concentrates in the heart and radiates out to the trunk.

In summary, under relationship stress, the visual loses perspective and can only see one point of view; the tonal hears what was never said or meant and picks up on a "vibe" that is often misinterpreted. The digital responds logically and rationally, despite a partner's request for feelings. And the kinesthetic is overwhelmed by emotions and lives in the moment, believing that feelings are facts.

Some of the **positives** of each sensory type are: **visuals** are visionaries, offer a compelling vision of what's possible, are persuasive, have strong convictions, and look you straight in the eye. **Tonals** are able to grasp and analyze a situation intuitively, are insightful, help you feel understood on many levels, and offer a nuanced and aesthetic sensitivity for matters that might go unnoticed by others. **Digitals** are kind and calm, have a systematic approach to life, are steady as a rock and unburdened by messy emotions, and have a gift for abstraction. **Kinesthetics** have the capacity for compassionately believing in others and knowing how they feel, are willing to sacrifice themselves for the other, and live each moment with true presence.

What happens when things get stressful? Visuals tell you how you "should" be, want to help you "get the picture," and expect you to appreciate how your life will improve if you just do what the visual says. The tonal hears between the lines inaccurately and doesn't understand the exact words but feels the tone, imagines accusations, feels insecurities, and experiences a cacophony of incoming experience. Digitals, believing they are totally right, offer solutions to problems when you just want to be heard, and are immune to others' feelings that just bounce off the digital, who creates a logical camouflage. Kinesthetics can implode with all the energies that are coming at them, are unable to think clearly, say yes to the wrong people for the wrong reason, are taken for granted, and can become a pushover. They cannot function well when they are accused, hurried, or pressured, and they lose their ability to express themselves in words.

Stop, Look, and Listen

What style do you think represents you? After reading the descriptions, does one type resonate with your perception of yourself? What's your predominant style when you are stressed or in conflict? Here is a practice you can use when experiencing relationship stress, a four-step process called a **Pact for Managing Conflict – Stop, Look, and Listen**. The **stop** component is two parts: stop the argument or conflict, and center your energies using the Blow Out (Expelling the Venom) from the 5 Rhythms exercises, the Neurovascular hold mentioned earlier, and the daily energy routine (from Chapter 5). This helps to calm things down, after which giving each other a spinal flush, which massages the neurolymphatic points alongside the spine, is a positive way to restore the connection between you. Doing a cross crawl (daily energy routine) or another activity together that helps energy to cross over will further the centering process and activate a positive bonding response.

For the **look** component, the point is to look with new eyes, beyond the limits of the type that you are, to really see your partner. When this is possible, you can return to the issue that is causing the conflict and use your typical survival mode *for* the relationship, first by checking out what your assumptions are (according to your typical reaction) and whether they truly reflect the truth of the matter. Once that is clarified, you can then respond in a way that takes into consideration the style of your partner so that the communication is balanced between both of your types.

A **visual** will express the partner's view of the circumstance, using their capacity for painting a compelling picture. A **tonal** will listen for the affirmative nuances in the partner's words and tone, drawing on the ability to hear the subtleties of words. A **digital** will have to stretch beyond the perception that they are right, and ask questions about what the partner's experience is, followed by the "Do you mean?'" technique to get clarification on an alternative possibility. By summarizing the partner's responses with empathy and caring, the digital shows understanding. A **kinesthetic** needs to ask the partner for what the kinesthetic needs right now, turning their strength for compassion toward themselves, and engaging the partner with this mindset.

The **listen** component starts with the **"Do you mean?" technique** for aligning your realities with each other, adjusted to your partner's style to maximize the potential for a positive outcome. The technique is used to determine if what you understand is correct regarding a statement that your partner has said, to which you ask, "Do you mean…?" Your partner responds with one of four possible answers: 1) Yes! (1 point), 2) No! (0 points), 3) part right, part wrong (1/2 point), and 4) I believe that to be true, but that is not what I was saying (0 points). Keep asking questions until you achieve 3 yeses. Once you have three yeses, you summarize with a statement:

> I can understand how [summary of what happened] would cause you to feel [name the feeling], and then ask for a confirmation that your partner feels you fully understand the initial statement, "Did I getcha?"

Another way of saying "Did I getcha?" is "Is there anything more?" and it is a vital element of the technique. It's designed to ensure that each incident is resolved as fully as possible because "for couples, what's not resolved will return" (Eden & Feinstein, 2014, p. 54). Once the partner who made the original statement feels understood, a statement of appreciation finishes off this part of the exchange and reinforces the success.

If at any time, you feel the conflict resurfacing, you can go back to stop and recenter your energies. **If your partner is visual**, look your partner straight in the eye, stand your ground, and let them see your eyes when you are being bullied, and don't expect a change in perspective during stress because they will need time to process. **If your partner is tonal**, listen to what is being said, acknowledge that you have heard your partner, and then help the tonal partner to check out the assumptions from "hearing between the lines."

If your partner is digital, don't expect a feeling response to an emotional matter and keep your own reaction cool and calm because if you raise your voice in frustration, that will turn off the digital partner. **If your partner is kinesthetic**, remove any pressure because your partner will not think clearly or function well when accused, hurried, or confronted with other's words or needs. Give plenty of time for your kinesthetic partner to process questions and requests, or they will only register your need, and take notice if your partner is suffering for you or unable to communicate.

No matter what type you are, genuine appreciation will transform the energy, so practice **"I appreciate"** at the end of the process, taking turns expressing the things you appreciate about your partner. You could also do some **"appreciation sandwiches,"** where you place your complaint or issue within two appreciations, which changes the context significantly.

Energy Check for Sensory Types

Finally, the way to **energy check, or test**, for sensory types is by using a general indicator test (the person extends their arm at shoulder height straightforward, and the tester applies pressure above the wrist for two seconds, creating a circuit with the other hand on the person's other shoulder; see photos 20 and 21) while the person being tested is thinking about a stress in their life. The person will **test strong** when looking in specific ways: the **visual test** has the person look the tester straight in the eye; the **tonal** will look down and to either side while being tested; the **digital** will look up and to the left when tested; and the **kinesthetic** looks straight down, so that they can stay with their own energies while being tested.

When you test strong for any of these, it is a good indication of what type you are. When I say test strong, it means the arm will stay up against any pressure. To work out your secondary type, you would think of a stressor that is less personal and test again, trying out all four possibilities. Then you will have both your primary and secondary sensory types. Know that sometimes when you are reacting to stress, it might be your secondary type that shows up and acts out. If you are aware of what it is, you can acknowledge that it is happening, and your partner will notice too. I highly recommend the book written by Donna Eden and David Feinstein, *The Energies of Love: Using Energy Medicine to Keep Your Relationship Thriving*

(2014). It will explain how the energetic dimensions of relationships play out and provide ideas for ways to work with those energies.

Knowing your rhythm and your sensory type gives you lots of information for how each of you plays your part in the relationship and how stress will impact on the connection. The stress of newborn parenting is enormous, so having a toolkit of strategies on hand that can alleviate the pressure is a powerful antidote to that stress. Although it has not been an emphasis in this chapter, neuroscience has been revealing the mechanisms by which we communicate with others, through resonance circuits that allow us to feel another person's feelings and create a cortical imprint for understanding what's going on in the other person's mind.

Daniel Siegel, whom we met in the Part on Bonding and Attachment, is the leader in the field of interpersonal neurobiology, and he calls this ability to appreciate the inner life of another the "mindsight mechanism." When we cannot identify with someone else, the resonance circuits shut down, and others become objects, which sets up a "them" and "us" polarity. The findings of these burgeoning fields throughout neuroscience are fascinating with what they uncover. Mindsight allows us to look deeply into the face of our partner and see the mind that exists beneath the surface through those mirror neurons. It may be another rhythm or another sensory type, but it is our beloved, and we resonate at levels that go very deep.

Summary for Nurturing Your Partner Relationship

I hope you will make an effort to remain lovers on this journey into parenthood, even when there might be a mismatch between your libido and your partner's. It is the magic that keeps you connected and teaches your child what love is all about. This quote from the book, *The Couple's Journey: Intimacy as a Path to Wholeness* (1980) by Susan Campbell, articulates how the relationship is transformative:

> The couple relationship may be the interpersonal unit most suited for transforming self and society to a new consciousness: a consciousness where interpersonal differences are seen as a source of learning and growth;

where conflicts between the individual and society can be negotiated from a dependable support base, and where the individual can experience human *interdependence* in a way that leads to seeing problems as the shared responsibility of all parts of the system (emphasis mine; Campbell, 1980, p. 181).

This Part has been a journey itself, through the discourse of relationship theory and practice, and energy approaches, over the last 50 years. It is my fervent desire that it helps you to make sense of how to remain present to your relationship as you expand your identities as parents and incorporate this new little being into your lives. Keep the conversations flowing when you falter through the minefield of newborn parenting, and you will emerge stronger, healthier, and more connected as a family.

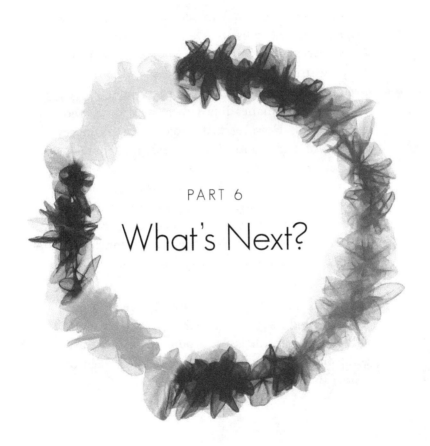

PART 6

What's Next?

PART 6 INTRODUCTION

What's next for most families emerging from the chrysalis of the postpartum period?

As I mentioned in the introduction, this chapter was originally meant to discuss *The Adverse Aftermath of Birth*, covering the unexpected consequences of birth, ranging from unplanned cesareans, birth trauma, perinatal mood and anxiety disorders, prematurity, congenital anomalies like Down syndrome, and perinatal loss. However, that "project" became more significant than I had anticipated and grew from one chapter into four. An agreement with my publisher was made to create a second book as a companion to this one that focuses on the adversity that some parents experience when they become parents. I will describe some of the important information that *The Adverse Aftermath of Birth* includes later in chapter 30.

When we made that decision, I realized there was one final issue: going back to work. This Part will engage with the issues around maternity leave, going back to work, and the policies that help or hinder this decision.

CHAPTER 28

Maternity Leave and Going Back to Work

Throughout the years that I ran groups and classes for new mothers and their babies, mothers frequently spoke of going back to work. Most of those years were in New York, although I did teach my mother and baby exercise class for a couple of years in the UK as well. Mothers in New York were grappling with so many aspects of the decision to go back to work. Should I go back to work? Should I not? Should it be full-time? Part-time? What options are there to change the work arrangements that are in place? If my organization is not flexible, should I look for a different job? Should I quit? Do I need to speak to my boss about these issues? Will I be able to manage the work/life balance of going back to work?

And then there is the issue of when to go back to work. American women do not get to stay home with their babies the way that British women can. Even the UK doesn't compare with other European nations that provide long paid maternity leave for mothers and paternity leave for fathers, especially in the more progressive Scandinavian countries. Living in the UK for 20 years, I've become accustomed to mothers having nine months to a year to spend with their babies before going back to work, even if it is not all paid, and the remuneration is low.

American Policy

Sadly, most American women are given only *six weeks* leave to spend with their babies before they are expected to return to work (8 weeks after a cesarean). And for many lower-income women, maternity leave is even shorter. That's wholly insufficient when you think that it takes that same six weeks just to recover from birth. Women can sometimes take an additional six weeks of "bonding time," but this may depend on which state you live in. None of it is paid. My daughter informed me of the policy in California, where she lives. When I Googled it, I found this:

> You may be entitled to *12 weeks* of job-protected leave *to bond* with your new baby. Male and female employees have the right to take bonding leave for up to 12 weeks to bond with a newborn baby, newly adopted or foster child (California Work and Family Coalition, 2012).

However, to be eligible for that, you need to work for a company that has at least 50 employees and have worked for the company for at least a year before taking the leave and working a minimum of 1,250 hours in that year. In October 2017, this was expanded for smaller-sized companies (with 20 to 49 employees) to provide 12 weeks of job-protected leave to bond with their newborns, a Parent Leave Act that was signed into law by Governor Brown on October 12, 2017.

California is one of five states (California, New Jersey, Rhode Island, New York, and Washington) where there are state laws protecting bonding leave, as well as the District of Columbia. Only three states—California, New Jersey, and Rhode Island—currently offer paid family and medical leave, and guarantee jobs when parents return from leave. The National Partnership for Women and Families has produced a great table on state leave laws which can be found at this link: http://www.nationalpartnership.org/research-library/work-family/paid-leave/state-paid-family-leave-laws.pdf. New York joins them effective Jan. 1, 2018, after passing the Paid Family Leave Benefits Law during the 2016 session. All four state programs are funded through employee-paid payroll taxes and administered through their respective disability programs (http://www.ncsl.org/research/labor-and-employment/state-family-and-medical-leave-laws.aspx).

As if 12 weeks is sufficient to bond with our babies; but something is better than nothing. It goes to show how different societies value the work of mothering and parenting. The United States is at the bottom of the list of industrialized countries for paid parental leave.

Denmark offers a year. Italy provides five months. France provides 16 weeks; Mexico, 12 weeks; Afghanistan, 13 [not even industrialized]. According to a 2016 Pew Research Center analysis of 41 countries, the U.S. is the only one to offer *zero paid* parental leave" (emphasis mine; Barron, 2017).

In Daniel Barron's blog, he reminds us of the enormous postpartum brain growth that is going on in the early weeks after birth, and that having leave to spend with the baby in these days and weeks is critical for how the brain will be sculpted, based on the interactions between parents and infants. With thousands of new synapses being created every day, those that are frequently used form networks of synaptic development, and those that aren't used are pruned and die off. Plain and simple: "Brain development is why the parent-child relationship is so important—you can keep an infant warm and nourished without it, but their brain won't develop properly" (Barron, 2017) This is a whole new take on the importance of paid family leave, and the author faces a paradox of being a resident in psychiatry and only having two weeks leave, not practicing the evidence-based science that they espouse to others. Barron sums it up nicely in this sentence: "Paid parental leave (for both parents) is associated with decreased infant mortality, less postpartum depression, more breastfeeding, more follow-up doctor appointments, and more involved dads—all things that promote healthy brain development" (Barron, 2017).

As for other states, in 2017, the state of Washington (one of the 5 states listed above) passed the most generous legislation for paid parental leave, but it doesn't start until 2020. For the time being, parents can fall back on family medical leave rights received under state and federal law for unpaid, but job-protected leave. This penchant for delaying the implementation of policy is part of Washington's history. Apparently, five weeks paid parental leave law was approved in 2007, but it's taken a decade for the funding component to be enacted, and in 2017, there is finally a funding plan and an implementation date. Come 2020, parents will have 12 weeks paid parental leave, and more if there is a family illness that requires extra time, and then an additional four weeks are available. This is both a parental leave and sick leave entitlement. For more information specific to Washington, this link will provide more details:

https://fairygodboss.com/career-topics/pregnancy-maternity-leave-and-paterni-ty-leave-in-washington-state.

Lactation-Accommodation Laws

While exploring what the maternity-leave positions were around the United States, I found that some things have improved over the years for breastfeeding women going back to work. There are now lactation-accommodation laws that require companies to provide time and space to express milk, as the quote below explains. After all, a generation of women who were determined to continue nursing after returning to work was forced to express their milk (and sometimes feed their babies) in bathroom cubicles. The California Work and Family Coalition have produced a document that sets out the laws that allow parents to nurture their child through bonding and breastfeeding, called "Six Key Laws for Parents." One of the California laws is for Lactation Accommodation and says, "Employed mothers have the right to break time and a private space to express breast milk for their babies."

> Federal and California State laws protect a woman's right to lactation accommodations. In California, all employers must provide breastfeeding mothers with break time and reasonable accommodations. The space should be private, free from intrusion, and in close proximity to the employee's work area. The lactation room *cannot be a bathroom stall.* Breastfeeding mothers can use their regular paid breaks. If an employed mother needs more time, employers must give them the additional break time, but it may be unpaid (emphasis mine; California Work and Family Coalition, 2012) http://paidfamilyleave.org/pdf/KeyLawPoster_ENG.pdf).

As is often the case, California was on the vanguard of accommodating nursing mothers returning to work, with their resolution that was passed in 1998 and signed into law in 2002 (Cal. Labor Code § 1030-1033) (England, 2017). This accommodation is mandatory for all employers, no matter what size the company. However, lactation accommodation was also codified in the Affordable Care Act in 2010, making it federal law as well, although this applies to organizations with 50 employees or more (Who knows what will happen with this acknowledgment of a mother's needs in the workplace with the evisceration of Obamacare by the current U.S. administration, along with women's reproductive rights in general. The federal law is called Section 7(r) of the Fair Labor Standards Act (FLSA): Break Time for Nursing Mothers Provision. This was an amendment to the FLSA law that was established in 1938. For those living in California (and other states), they are protected by this clause: "Nothing in this subsection shall preempt a State law that provides greater protections to employees than the protections provided for under this subsection," says the Department of Labor (U.S. Department of Labor, Wage and Hour Division, n.d.b). For American mothers who want to learn more about their rights in this regard, this link will take you to the federal page that provides all the information (as of 2017), which we can only hope will be updated: (U.S. Department of Labor, Wage and Hour Division, n.d.). https://www.dol.gov/whd/nursingmothers/.

The state of New York passed Section 206-c of the New York State Labor Law, "requiring all public and private employers, regardless of the size or nature of their business, to provide nursing mothers with unpaid breaks, or paid break or meal times, to express breast milk" (Lawyers Alliance, 2009). It also applies to all sized employers and continues for up to three years. The "Guidelines Regarding the Rights of Nursing Mothers to Express Breast Milk in the Work Place" was written in 2008, to help employers interpret the law that went into effect in 2007 (New York State Labor Law, 2009). New York was ahead of the federal government with this law, in a similar fashion to the New York state law that went into effect in 1970 that legalized abortion, which then became federal law in 1973 with the Supreme Court Roe v Wade decision that legalized abortion nationally.

In New Jersey, their maternity leave is embedded in their Family Leave Act, which combines both bonding leave and care for a family member. Their Family Leave Insurance (FLI) program provides up to 6 weeks of partially paid maternity leave under the Temporary Disability Benefits Law. Temporary Disability Insurance (TDI) covers a portion of lost wages for women who are unable to work due to medical complications related to their pregnancy or childbirth, typically beginning four weeks before delivery through six weeks after birth (eight after a cesarean section). This can be extended if there were complications that a doctor certifies indicating the woman is unable to physically perform the job.

Most New Jersey employees are eligible for FLI for the time when they wish to bond with their newborn or adopted child. FLI benefits are entirely employee-funded, through a small portion of their paychecks withheld for all NJ employees earning over a certain limit to pay for the benefits. However, FLI does not protect a woman's job, so New Jersey passed the New Jersey Family Leave Act (NJFLA) that requires employers to provide up to 12 weeks of unpaid family leave that protects the job while employees are gone. Similar to the federal Family Leave Act, the NJFLA applies to more people because it includes employers who have 50 or more global employees (instead of the federal requirement that they be within a 75-mile radius). Eligibility depends on working at a company for at least 12 months and clocking a minimum of 1,000 hours. The NJFLA applies to private and public employers and prohibits discrimination against women due to pregnancy and birth-related conditions. Although employers may not treat pregnant women less favorably and it provides reasonable accommodations like bathroom breaks and assistance with manual labor, it doesn't mention anything about lactation accommodation (Fairygodboss, n.d.).

Twenty states, plus the District of Columbia and Puerto Rico, have Workplace Breastfeeding Rights, and those can be found at this website: https://www.dol.gov/wb/maps/4.htm. Some rights have been mitigated – e.g., in Georgia, employers are allowed, but not required, to provide time and space for expressing milk. In Mississippi, the policy says they cannot forbid breastfeeding. In Louisiana, only employees of public schools have these rights (what's that about?). You can find out the statutes for each state on Workplace Breastfeeding Rights through that link.

Pregnancy and Maternity Discrimination

The incidence of pregnancy discrimination has been highlighted over the last decade, and it's a subject that goes far beyond the remit for this chapter. When my daughter was pregnant with her second child, she experienced pregnancy discrimination by her boss at her job. Eventually, she did bring a grievance claim against him, and he was pushed out of his position. But the experience was so negative that she decided not to go back to work there. Below is a link to a website that informs women when to consider hiring a lawyer if they are experiencing pregnancy discrimination. Here's what the author, Deborah C. England, describes about discrimination when going back to work:

> If your employer interferes with your return from leave, your attorney can assess whether the interference is discriminatory. For example, if your employer does indeed replace you with the "temp" hired to fill in during your leave, you may want your lawyer to contact your employer and ask about the status of your job. If your employer can't give a convincing reason as to why you were replaced, you'll probably have solid grounds for a pregnancy discrimination claim (England, *Pregnancy Discrimination: When You Should Talk to a Lawyer*: https://www.nolo.com/legal-encyclopedia/pregnancy-discrimination-when-you-should-talk-lawyer.html).

Knowing your rights is critical. The Legal Aid at Work organization has lots of information about maternity rights in the workplace, including many fact sheets, and a Work and Family helpline: **415-593-0033 or 800-800-8047.** Based in San Francisco, Legal Aid at Work has written a 6-page fact sheet called *Taking Leave from Work: Pregnancy/Prenatal Care/ Bonding with a New Child* that explains everything you want to know about disability leave, bonding leave, and other rights in California, including lactation accommodations: https://legalaidatwork.org/our-programs/work-and-family-program/. I can imagine that there are organizations like this in many states, not just California, and it's worth investigating them while you are considering under what circumstances you want to go back to work. At the moment, San Francisco has the strongest accommodation law in the U.S.

To Work or Not to Work?

Some mothers will decide that they don't want to go back to work at all. They may be in a position that makes this possible if their partner is earning enough income to support the family, or they are just going to take some time off with their babies before looking for a new job. There is a lot of pressure on stay-at-home mothers to "do" something in the labor force, a remnant of the feminist movement. Some mothers feel the need to justify their choice to stay at home with their children. What I observed with the mothers in my groups and classes was when the first child was born their identity was more wrapped up in their job experience than with motherhood. No one pats you on the back for changing diapers/nappies or breastfeeding your baby, but there is lots of recognition for achievements in the workplace. The unpaid labor of motherhood can feel like a thankless task. So, they go back to work, where there are adults they can talk to, and give them acknowledgment of their successes.

However, when their second child comes along, they've been a mother long enough for that to be an integrated part of their expanded identity. Then, they feel able to make the decision to stay home as a mother, and it helps that they are experienced in being a mother over a period of time. The potential chaos and turbulence in the weeks and months after a first child is born can be an incentive to going back to work. With subsequent children, that's history, and life after birth can be orderly and calm for experienced parents, making it easier to make different choices that enable staying home as an empowered decision. The Mommy Wars, where stay-at-home moms and career moms face off with each other, speak to the attitudes of those who believe that women should take part in the labor force and those who choose to stay home with children. Often, this involves second thoughts about the decision they made, as they question what's right for their children and themselves. The Mommy Wars concept may be overstated, but for generations, there have been differences in how mothers viewed their participation in the labor market once second-wave feminists succeeded in getting women into the workforce in the second half of the 20th century.

Childcare

Going back to work means finding childcare while you're at work. You can choose a daycare center, family daycare, someone who takes children into their home (in England, it's called a childminder), or a nanny who works in your home. This will be only a brief discussion about childcare, because I don't want to make the same mistake of turning a chapter into a book, as childcare issues warrant a full book, and I'm sure those have been written. It's hard to know what the best option for us is. Some people don't want someone coming into their home, and when they do hire someone, they can be concerned about the need for surveillance. My daughter had a very successful experience with a nanny who stayed with her for five ½ years until both children were in school, and there were no such concerns.

There are those that send their children to a family daycare center but wonder about the quality of care they receive. Although it was for just one day a week, I sent my youngest to a family daycare home to have some time to myself and some social experience for him. The thing that annoyed me was how quickly colds would pass from one child to another, though that is not specific to family daycare. It can happen in daycare centers too. Daycare centers come in all shapes and sizes, and quality can vary from place to place. However, they have the advantage of structured learning experiences and social development.

Unfortunately, what often happens is that all or most of the income a mother earns can end up paying just for daycare. In this case, it would be important to evaluate the benefits and risks of that. A family member decided it wasn't worth paying the fees once her second child was born, and the costs of care for two children became totally prohibitive. If you are not able to use the money you earn because it all goes to daycare, is it worth it to be away from your baby for long days? It can be, if a woman feels passionately about her work, and it's more than just the money.

Maternity-Leave Registry

I read an online article presenting a great idea for arranging more time to be home with your baby: a maternity-leave registry. It is literally the gift of time, in which you can Crowdfund for leave time. The article by Michelle Woo highlights how 25% of women are forced to return to work at *two weeks* postpartum. A platform was created for this purpose by Take12, a maternity-leave registry, and here is what the article said:

> A platform created for this purpose is **Take12**, a maternity-leave registry. It's pretty straightforward—instead of asking your pals to buy you onesies or bibs or that $25 rubber giraffe, you register for the "gift of time." Those

who visit your customized site can give money to cover the various moments of maternity leave—snuggles, shower time for Mom, a night of sleep…Your friends and family may only be able to cover a tiny portion of that, but the point of the registry is also to "elevate the importance of sufficient family leave." Of course, if we're making a statement, dads should be included, too. A stigma exists for many fathers when it comes to taking paternity leave, even when the benefits are evident (https://offspring. lifehacker.com/this-maternity-leave-registry-site-lets-you-crowdfund-t-1818502196).

Although some initial reactions to this idea of crowdfunding for leave have been critical (seemingly tacky), I think it's a wonderful idea for new parents. It does require that all the costs, not only lost income, are covered, such as birth expenses, life insurance, support services (doulas or lactation consultants), and baby goods.

CHAPTER 29

Government and Employer Policies Around the World

Before we move on to policies from other parts of the world, I was reminded that it's important to know that employers will have their own policies for maternity leave wherever you live. In the United States, there are many companies, mainly in Corporate America, that have excellent policies for their employees. It can be a very different experience for people who work in small businesses that don't have any policy at all. I can remember about 35 years ago, I had a client who worked for *Working Woman* magazine (which ceased publication after 25 years in 2001), which ironically did not have a maternity-leave policy. How crazy is that? I was surprised to read an online article about the 19 U.S. companies with the best policies for parental leave and other perks that go with the job, ranging from 12 weeks paid leave to a full year, in *19 Companies and Industries with Radically Awesome Parental Leave Policies*. Although its date is April 2017, it talks about Mark Zuckerberg having his first child, so parts of it were probably gathered a while ago. Here's the link to see what's on offer: https://www.entrepreneur.com/slideshow/249467 (Entrepreneur, 2017).

What happens to those who work for companies without a policy for parental leave? In conversations with a colleague in Australia, she told me that when she took her leave, she wasn't able to receive any assistance. Her company had no policy, and she was over the threshold for receiving government leave (in Australia, that cutoff is $150,000). I'm imagining this is true in many countries around the world, where parents can slip through the net by circumstances. This information is not well-published, but in Australia, which is detailed down below, the range can be from nothing to six weeks on the low end, to 3 to 12 months paid leave with more progressive and modern companies. Employers are evolving with the times, and hopefully, this trend of offering more leave and benefits will continue in recognition of the needs of childbearing women and their families.

British Policy

One way the UK has as an advantage over the U.S. is that the UK has a national policy. States may have their own rules that sometimes conflict with the federal ones. There may be differences between countries within the UK, but they will still be national policies. Scotland has devolved a lot of its political control, and England and Wales often go together when it comes to policy. Statutory Maternity Leave for eligible employees allows up to *52 weeks maternity leave.* The first 26 weeks is known as "Ordinary Maternity Leave," and the last 26 weeks as "Additional Maternity Leave." The earliest that leave can be taken is 11 weeks before the expected week of childbirth, unless the baby is born early. Eligibility depends on the person working for at least 26 weeks continuous employment by the 15th week before the expected due date (https://www.gov.uk/maternity-pay-leave). You can see what a difference it makes to have 52 weeks over 12 weeks.

When it comes to paid leave, here is what's available: Statutory Maternity Pay (SMP) for eligible employees can be paid for up to 39 weeks, usually as follows: the first 6 weeks: 90% of their average weekly earnings (AWE) before tax. The remaining 33 weeks: a flat rate of 140.98£ per week (April 2017 - April 2018; this adjusts from year to year), or 90% of their AWE (whichever is lower). The employer pays your SMP in the same way as your salary is paid. So, British women have paid leave for 75% of a full year. To me, that is a much more humane approach to new mothers and employment rights.

In April 2015, Shared Parental Leave (SPL) went into effect, allowing employed parents to share time in caring for their babies in the first year after birth. The mother must take at least two weeks of maternity leave immediately after birth, and they can share the remaining 50 weeks. There is also Shared Parental Pay (ShPP), paid in the same way once maternity leave pay has ended. So, if a woman takes 12 weeks of maternity leave, the couple can share the remaining 40 weeks of leave, and 37 weeks of parental pay.

However, what became apparent once this system was in place was that most families are unable to support themselves on the meager £140.98 a week or less that shared parental pay offers. While it is good to have a policy in principle, there is a real issue of it being financially unworkable, and some mothers are not willing to give up their leave to have shared leave. In a recent study, 50% of men felt that taking leave would damage their career and only 1% had applied for it (Kemp, 2016). It is anticipated that more will take advantage of shared parental leave as more people become aware of its existence, and a shift in attitudes about what men have to sacrifice to take that time off in the way of career aspirations. For more specific details of SPL, check out the UK government website: https://www.gov.uk/shared-parental-leave-and-pay.

Maternity Discrimination

A research project into maternity discrimination was commissioned in 2015 by the Department for Business, Innovation, and Skills (BIS) and the Equality and Human Rights Commission (EHRC). They found that maternity discrimination is widespread and has worsened dramatically in the past 10 years. Each year, 54,000 women lose their job as a result of maternity discrimination, an 80% increase since 2005, when an Equal Opportunities Commission research project was undertaken. The Women and Equalities Select Committee of the House of Commons produced the 71-page report on *Pregnancy and Maternity Discrimination* (2016), on how many more women are being made redundant or feel forced to leave their job. Another shocking finding was that more than three quarters (77%) of the women surveyed had experienced a negative or potentially discriminatory experience as a result of their pregnancy or maternity. Once the government uncovered the scale of discrimination, they had to ascertain what the next steps are for the protection of women's maternity rights, with input from many organizations (House of Commons Women and Equalities Select Committee, 2016). In this document, the "Rights of All Employees and Workers" assures protection from discrimination:

16. All women are entitled to protection from discrimination by their employer because of their pregnancy or maternity. Under the Equality Act 2010, it is unlawful for an employer to discriminate against a woman because of her pregnancy, pregnancy-related sickness, or maternity leave. Discriminatory treatment can include dismissal, redundancy, removal of responsibilities, denial of a bonus, and being overlooked for promotion. Some forms of harassment may also be classed as sex discrimination.

Another section of the report includes "rest facilities," which approximates but doesn't go as far as providing lactation accommodation:

19. Employers are required to provide suitable rest facilities for all pregnant and breastfeeding workers, but there is no legal duty to provide a place to breastfeed or store milk.

Maternity Action

One of the many organizations that contributed to the House of Commons report is Maternity Action, the leading UK charity whose mission is to end inequality and improve the health and wellbeing of pregnant women, partners, and young children, from conception through the child's early years (www.maternityaction.org.uk). They offer free advice on work and benefits, National Health Service (NHS) maternity care, and advice and training for health professionals and other community workers involved in migrant women's care. They have a comprehensive page on Shared Parental Leave, covering everything you'd need to know, on their website (Maternity Action, n.d.).

Maternity Action also convenes the *Alliance for Maternity Rights*, a coalition including unions and parents' organizations that collaborate on making policy recommendations to eliminate pregnancy and maternity discrimination and achieve fairness for pregnant and new mothers. The Alliance successfully lobbied the Government to undertake research into maternity discrimination at work, running campaigns to end pregnancy discrimination in the UK. Most recently, Maternity Action produced a report on *Unfair Redundancies: During Pregnancy, Maternity Leave and*

Return to Work (Maternity Action, 2017). Redundancy in the UK refers to the loss of a job because the job no longer exists, or the role is no longer required. It is extremely difficult to make someone on maternity leave redundant, but apparently, this still takes place. Hence, the report on its incidence.

I was made redundant when my fixed-term contracts ended on a couple of positions I held as an academic health researcher. The October 2017 report called on the government to act on its commitment to review redundancy protection, made earlier in January 2017 but not acted on. It found that about 1 in 20 mothers (6%) were made redundant during pregnancy, maternity leave, or return to work. Much of this report is based on the Parliamentary report just discussed and includes many case studies of women's actual experience with discrimination and redundancies. They recommend adopting the German model of redundancy protection: where women must not be made redundant from the time they notify a pregnancy through the six months after return to work, with some limited exceptions. There are a total of 12 recommendations for forward action in the Maternity Action report on unfair redundancies.

In the UK, maternity leave is generous compared to the U.S., with paid leave for 75% of the first year after birth and shared parental leave for parents that encourages fathers to be involved with their children's care and development.

French Policy

I was lucky to have a client who lives in France while I was compiling the data on maternity leave, and she was able to collate some information for me on how maternity leave works in France. There were some surprises when I tuned in to what the policy actually is, and what is provided for mothers and fathers. Paternity leave is for 11 consecutive days: *Saturday, Sunday, and public holidays included* (Amelie.fr for the insured, 2017). It increases to 18 days if there are multiple births. I think this bespeaks a level of patriarchy in lawmakers' attitudes regarding which parent should be doing the parenting, ignoring the importance of paternal involvement. I was also surprised to learn that France only offers 16 weeks of paid maternity leave for first and second babies, and it's broken down into prenatal, 6 weeks, and postnatal, 10 weeks. It is mandatory for a mother to take at least 8 weeks leave. Sometimes, if the mother is in good health, which must be certified by a physician, she can arrange to have more time after birth by having less before birth:

> To give more freedom to women whose pregnancy is going well and allow them to spend more time with their baby, the terms of maternity leave have been relaxed: you can ask to postpone part of your prenatal leave (the first 3 weeks maximum) on your postnatal leave. This report can be done with the agreement of your doctor:
>
> ▶ in one go for a maximum of 3 weeks;
>
> ▶ either in the form of a postponement of a duration fixed by your doctor and renewable (one or more times) within the limit of 3 weeks.
>
> The steps to be taken: Send a written request to your health insurance fund, accompanied by a certificate from your doctor or midwife attesting that your state of health allows you to extend your professional activity before birth. You must apply no later than 1 day before the originally scheduled date of your leave (https://www.ameli.fr/assure/droits-demarches/famille/maternite-paternite-adoption/conge-maternite).

How much time a mother is given for maternity leave changes when there are more children in the family or with multiple births:

> Your maternity leave includes prenatal leave (before delivery) and postnatal leave (after childbirth). Its legal duration, set by the Social Security Code and the Labor Code varies according to the number of children you expect and the number of children you have already had (https://www.ameli.fr/assure/droits-demarches/famille/maternite-paternite-adoption/conge-paternite-accueil-enfant).

The amount of paid weeks of maternity leave depends on your situation:

- ▶ 16 weeks if this is your first or second child,
- ▶ 26 weeks if this is your third child,
- ▶ 34 weeks if you are expecting twins, or
- ▶ 46 weeks if you are expecting triplets or more

http://frenchmamma.com/maternity-leave-france/.

Reading through all the data on French maternity leave, I found the bureaucracy of it daunting. When a woman becomes pregnant, she needs to register with both her health professional and her local health insurance fund, where she can get advice and information on pregnancy and birth-related costs, and her entitlement for paid leave. Health insurance in France pays 100% of all expenses.

> Following your first antenatal examination (*premier examen prénata*), which must be before the end of the third month, you will be given a three-page document declaring your pregnancy in France (*declaration de grossesse*). You will need this to claim health insurance for childbirth in France and social security coverage for parental leave in France (Expatica, 2016) (https://www.expatica.com/fr/healthcare/Having-a-baby-in-France_107664.html).

> …To qualify for parental leave in France you must have worked at least 150 hours within a period of three months, or 600 hours within 12 months if working part-time or sporadically. There are other ways to qualify, although you typically don't need to do anything to receive your benefit; your health insurer will assess your eligibility and send a salary certificate to your employer outlining what you will get … New mothers and fathers on parental leave in France receive a daily benefit equal to their average wage during the three-month period before the birth in France, up to the monthly social security ceiling of EUR 3,218 monthly (2016)…subject to yearly change (Expatica, 2016).

On both government websites and others that I've read, there is so much detail to work through and so many rules to follow, that it brings new meaning to French bureaucracy. I have quoted so extensively from the websites because I wanted to be sure I articulated accurately what's involved. However, I learned so much about how the system works, and how insurance run by the state has very different outcomes than insurance companies running the medical system as they do in the U.S. I hadn't known France had a third-party system of coverage for medical expenses and benefits. It seems that "Your French health insurer" is an integrated part of the health care system, and not as profit-driven as health insurance in the U.S. Instead, it works hand in hand with the government in the delivery of services. Maternity and paternity insurance assures that parents have paid leave and all birth-related costs are covered, at no expense to the family. Here is how it is explained:

> As from January 1st, 2017, the third-party payment system applies to all medical care that is covered by the maternity-insurance system at a rate of 100% and provided by non-hospital-based health professionals. This means that the patient does not pay for any care upfront as *Assurance Maladie* pays the healthcare professional directly for the appointment or procedures performed (http://www.cleiss.fr/docs/regimes/regime_france/an_1.html).

The French Labor Code has laws against pregnancy discrimination (http://www.equineteurope.org/DescriptionAn-awareness-raising) that are influenced by the European Union, and also the European Court of Human Rights, established in 1959 as a judicial body guaranteeing the rights enshrined in the European Convention on Human Rights, for everyone living in one of the 47 contracting states. One wonders if women living in France have to fight against discrimination in the way women in the U.S. and the UK do. In the next section, we can see how maternity leave works in another English-speaking country.

Australian Policy

To start off, under the Fair Work Act in Australia, new parents can take a 12-month unpaid parental leave, and parents can request another 12 months leave if the employer agrees. You have to have been employed for 12 months to be eligible. It's a generous amount of leave time, but how many people can afford to go without income for that length of time? The Fair Work Commission tackles issues of discrimination and other reasons for dismissal, and there are 21 days to lodge an application with the Commission for help in resolving workplace issues (Australian Government Fair Work Ombudsman, n.d.).

Parents are entitled to their pre-leave job back, or another available position they are qualified for, and nearest in pay and status to the pre-leave job if it no longer exists, which is the "return to work guarantee" (Supporting Working Parents, 2015a). Breastfeeding is considered a "protected ground of discrimination" (Supporting Working Parents, 2015b), and women can request a private room with a comfortable chair, a fridge to store breast milk and somewhere to store a breast pump. "Failure to provide adequate facilities may constitute discrimination and a breach of work health and safety laws" (Supporting Working Parents, 2015b).

However, reading further, I learned that there is Paid Parental Leave if you meet specific criteria, such as a work test that indicates employment for at least 13 months before the leave, in which you have worked for 10 of those months; residence requirements for the duration of paid leave; adjusted taxable income at $150,000 or below; and of course, being the person responsible for primary care of the new baby or adopted child. This was the only country that stipulated an income cutoff among all I reviewed. The Australian Paid Parental Leave scheme, introduced in 2011, provides paid parental leave but doesn't give an entitlement to leave. Apparently, the Fair Work Act and Paid Parental Leave program have different eligibility criteria, the former being about leave entitlement and the latter about payment for leave. Maternity pay is for 18 weeks at the national minimum wage, which works out to $695 a week and is taxable. Dad and Partner pay is for two weeks at the same rate (Australian Department of Human Services, 2017).

What I found interesting is the implied assumption that the recipient of parental leave is the mother, and I wasn't able to ascertain if there was something called paternity leave. When the name changes to parental leave, I always think that's because it includes leave for the father or partner as well. Why change the name if it's maternity leave for all intents and purposes? I trawled through many websites trying to find paternity leave and didn't see it, even when I checked the link: "Dad and Partner Pay does not change *leave entitlements* and your partner should check with their employer as to what leave they are entitled to" (emphasis mine; The Bub Hub Crew, 2017). This statement corroborates my comment that it's the mother who's being addressed. And it appeared that if there is leave entitlement, it's up to the employer to determine it. But I was wrong.

After doggedly persisting in looking for paternal leave, I found that fathers are also entitled to 12 months unpaid parental leave (which was worded to include same-sex couples), and that it can be taken in a number of ways. Either it can be one parent taking leave, or both can take leave; it can be at different times in the first year or concurrently, and for either parent, it must be taken in a single continuous period. When both parents take leave at the same time, they can take up to 8 weeks unpaid parental leave, or concurrent leave. It is considered part of an employee's total unpaid parental-leave entitlement and will be deducted from the total entitlement. Concurrent leave can be taken in separate periods, but each needs to be at least two weeks long. When leave is taken at different times, they can take up to 12 months, but the combined leave can't be longer than 24 months. Leave would begin on the date of birth or adoption placement, although the pregnant woman can take up to six weeks before the due date. It still works as one continuous period so one parent would have to begin their unpaid leave the next working day after the first parent's leave ends (https://www.fairwork.gov.au/leave/maternity-and-parental-leave/taking-parental-leave). To sum up parental leave in Australia, it is a generous period of unpaid leave for both parents, of which mothers receive Paid Parental Leave for 18 weeks, and fathers for 2 weeks.

Around the World

What about the rest of the world? We hear so much about Scandinavian countries, which were on the vanguard of providing leave for generations, but these days, some countries have improved on those longstanding patterns. At this website on maternity leave around the world (http://www.instantoffices.com/blog/featured/maternity-leave-around-world/), I learned that Croatia and Serbia have joined the ranks of high-quality leave and benefits for families. I imagine that their recent re-establishment as sovereign countries was an opportunity to put good policies into law. Sweden and Norway are also incorporated by tradition, and the UK is included, but some of the information is not accurate, so we always have to be careful about information that appears on the internet.

According to the infographic, Sweden is at the top of countries with the most maternity leave, offering 480 days at 80% of the current salary, provided by social insurance (tax paid). #2 is Croatia, with 365+ days at 100% of wages paid, provided by health insurance funds. Next is Norway, between 322 to 365 days at 80-100%, also with social insurance. #4 is the UK, but it says the 365 days are paid at 90%, but that's only for the first six weeks of statutory maternity pay, or when that 90% is below the £140.98 flat rate for the duration). The remaining 33 weeks is the flat rate of £140.98. The last of the five on this list is Serbia, offering 365 days at 100% paid wages, provided by social security, but when you look closer that 100% is for the first 26 weeks, 60% at 27 to 39 weeks, and 30% for the remaining weeks of the year.

If we look at the fine print, there we find the specifics for each country. Sweden has the most progressive working environments and benefits, and paid parental leave can be shared by the parents as 240 days each as the country strives for gender equality. Sweden also provides 90 days of personal leave for each parent, exclusively for him or her, and parents can shorten their work weeks by 25% until the child turns 8. Parents can take parental leave until the child turns 8, and this leave accumulates when there are more children in the family. In Croatia, where the mother can receive 100% paid maternal leave for a year, it also says, "Aside from a year of bonding with the new-born, full paid parental leave is available for 120 days" (http://www.instantoffices.com/blog/featured/maternity-leave-around-world/). I'm really not sure what that means, or if it refers to the partner, because the leave focuses on the mother. Apparently, Croatia is very protective of mothers with laws in place that provide free antenatal and postnatal care, one-hour breastfeeding breaks until the child turns one, protection from dismissal during pregnancy and maternity leave, the right to return to the same job after leave, and pregnant and nursing mothers don't have to do harmful work. There are other flexible options when there are children who have exceptional needs and for parents of all minors. Norway "is regarded as a *mastermind* when it comes to understanding the real implications of a work-life balance, and for such a small country, the participation of women in the workforce is crucial" (Instant Offices, 2017). Parents get 46 weeks of 100% full salary or 56 weeks at 80% pay. Dedicated to reducing the gender pay gap and the motherhood penalty, Norway has the second highest male-to-female earned income, depending on what your source is. Iceland is the first, and Finland and Norway are ranked next (http://reports.weforum.org/global-gender-gap-report-2016/rankings/). Norway also advocates for shorter working days for parents, and yet has very high productivity, intent on attaining a successful work/life balance. And fathers are essential partners in parenting in Norway:

> The culture of equality in Norway is evident in the country's efforts to make fathers feel like they're playing an active parental role, rather than acting as additional caregivers in the family. It's common for male employees to reschedule meetings with colleagues to allow for commitments like school concerts, sports games, or simply wanting to collect kids from school at a reasonable hour.

> Another way of treating fathers as equals in Norwegian culture is the policy that states that if fathers don't take their share of paternal leave, then the total parental leave is shortened. This encourages fathers to bond with their children and support their early development while motivating mothers to go back to work. It's a win-win-win (Instant Offices, 2017).

The data on the UK is unreliable, but this article does raise the issue of how little paternity leave fathers actually take. It's almost the antithesis of Norway. Despite shared parental leave, in 2012, fathers only took an average of 9.39 days; in 2013, 9.57 days; and in 2014, it rose to 12.22 days. As I mentioned above, there is a stigma against fathers taking time off in the UK. And finally, Serbia has some rules about maternity leave that are confusing. Here's what this article says regarding leave:

- starts no earlier than 45 days before the due date
- begins no later than 28 days before the due date
- lasts for three months from the date of birth
- is fully paid by the state
- can be taken for up to 20 weeks, fully paid, after giving birth (Instant Offices, 2017)

I wonder if it's for 3 months or 20 weeks, but then it says that "after that, mothers qualify for an additional full year of leave, with compensation lowering over time," as I described above. Mothers' jobs are protected, and they cannot be fired during pregnancy and maternity leave. However, paternal leave is for one fully-paid week only.

There's a lot of diversity in the different arrangements that these top five countries offer in the way of parental leave. Doing the research for this entire section of the chapter really opened my eyes to the rules and regulations that parents must navigate when it comes to going back to work. Among rankings for the global gender-pay gap, the UK is #20, the US is #45, and Australia is #46 (http://reports.weforum.org/global-gender-gap-report-2016/rankings/). Rwanda is #5. There is still work to be done for equal pay worldwide, but that's another book. I tried to find a graphic to finish off this section, but those I could find were so inconsistent, in terms of which countries were included, that I decided against it. In the next chapter, I will explain more about the companion book to this one that grew out of the development of *Life After Birth: A Parent's Holistic Guide for Thriving in the Fourth Trimester*. We expect it will be published shortly after this one.

CHAPTER 30

The Adverse Aftermath of Birth

While I was writing this book over a number of years, I became acutely aware that not everyone has the positive experience with new parenting that I have been encouraging throughout this book, and it was essential to address their needs too. I had a postnatal doula client whose baby was premature, born at 29 weeks, and spent the first eight weeks of his life in the Neonatal Intensive Care Unit (NICU). Hers was undoubtedly not the kind of experience that we've been discussing in this book, and it became clear that other circumstances would challenge parents' capacity in the weeks and months after birth. What about parents who are depressed or anxious? What about women who've had an unplanned cesarean section? What about the countless women and their partners who emerge from their birth experience feeling traumatized? Or women who have other mental health problems? Then there are parents of babies who have congenital anomalies like Down syndrome or birth defects. And perinatal loss is devastating, though it's highly unlikely that those parents will be reading books on the postpartum period. Who's speaking for these new parents? I felt I had a duty to address their adverse aftermath of birth.

Back in the summer of 2017, when I was writing the chapter that was going to be called the "Adverse Aftermath of Birth," the content of this chapter cum section cum new book kept growing exponentially. There was so much to say on all the many unexpected challenges that can arise after birth, and this was a function of the work that I have been doing over the last few years advocating for changes in perinatal mental health and infant mental health services. As a member of the All-Party Parliamentary Group (APPG) for Conception to Age 2: the first 1001 days, I've had the privilege of working alongside other advocates and experts on this subject in regular meetings in the House of Commons. This also resulted in my contributing a chapter on birth trauma (Speier, 2017) in *Transforming Infant Wellbeing: Research, Policy, and Practice for the First 1001 Critical Days*, edited by Penelope Leach. After weeks of writing and synthesizing so much relevant material, the next book breaks down into the following sections, all of which continue to offer Eden Energy Medicine techniques for managing the various situations.

1. When the Unexpected Happens – Surgery and Trauma

This section covers how the advent of various diagnostic tests and screening can sometimes raise their own issues with false positive (erroneously saying there is a problem) and false negative (wrongly saying there isn't a problem when one exists) results, questioning their reliability in foreseeing any complications. Then there is the loss of a dream when the unexpected happens, with an in-depth examination of unplanned cesareans and birth trauma. The cesarean section chapter involves recovery from a surgical delivery, complications, breastfeeding, and what the risks and causes are of cesarean sections. The trauma chapter is a comprehensive exploration of causes, risks, treatments, and prevention. There are also personal vignettes of two women's experiences after birth trauma and how it impacted on their lives.

2. Perinatal Depression and Anxiety

This section is about depression and anxiety that often starts during the prenatal period, which often predicts whether someone will have postpartum depression and/or anxiety. When this happens during pregnancy, it also has an impact on the fetus and its development. Perinatal mental illness is the most common complication of birth, affecting up to 20% of women. This chapter invites the reader to consider a new paradigm of depression that is based on the inflammatory response, grounded in new research that demonstrates how inflammation contributes to depressive illness and other chronic diseases. Many holistic strategies can help going beyond antidepressant treatment, such as psychotherapy, mindfulness, nutrition and supplements, exercise and yoga, lots of body contact with our babies, and breastfeeding. Seeking help and a variety of resources for those who suffer are also presented, along with another vignette from a mother who experienced depression and anxiety.

Paternal postpartum depression is also addressed as we learn more about how fathers are affected, how gender roles play out in the transition to fatherhood, and the impact this has on the partner relationship and the bond with the baby. It finishes with another vignette, this time from a father who experienced depression after the births of his children.

3. Psychosis, Bipolar Disorder, and OCD

This section goes into the more severe and enduring types of mental illnesses that are caused by birth, or conditions that are exacerbated by the pregnancy for those with pre-existing conditions. Puerperal (postpartum) psychosis is the most severe illness among the perinatal mood and anxiety disorders, thankfully happening in only one or two women out of a thousand. There is a list of services that include Mother and Baby Units (MBU) in the UK, the U.S., and Australia as the main focus. The vignette of a woman's journey through psychosis beautifully illustrates this descent into madness and the return to normality thanks to an MBU offering her care.

Bipolar disorder is often diagnosed for the first time after a woman has a baby, and this usually requires the use of medication to manage mood swings, but other holistic strategies are presented too, especially nutritional therapy. I found it so interesting that the academic literature on bipolar disorder mainly concerned managing the symptoms, but did not explain what it was, while the nutrition therapy/alternative route gave highly detailed interpretations of what's happening.

The final part is on obsessive-compulsive disorder (OCD), and the paralyzing effects it can have on a mother and her relationship with her baby because it impairs functionality. The vignette for this section tells the story of a woman who had miscarried in her first pregnancy and how this affected her next pregnancy and the years after, a long journey not yet resolved.

4. Prematurity and Congenital Abnormalities

This section discusses prematurity and the impact this has on the parents, especially the mother, when the baby needs to spend a protracted amount of time being cared for by NICU staff. Parenting feels tentative in those early weeks. The story of my client, who I opened this chapter with, is included for a deeper understanding of what prematurity involves, and the challenges that this entails for parents.

The second part of this chapter examines what happens to parents who give birth to babies who have congenital anomalies, like Down syndrome, and other birth defects. The vignette for this section involves a mother who gave birth to a son with Down syndrome without any advanced warning (she did not have an amniocentesis). This mom has been grappling with various other medical conditions that her son has faced in the years since his birth.

5. Perinatal Loss

This section covers the issues of miscarriage, stillbirth, and infant death, and specific perinatal losses that parents suffer, with the more serious ones having a devastating effect on parents. This often has a damaging impact on future pregnancies, often resulting in trauma that carries through subsequent pregnancies. Contrary to the myth that a healthy baby will resolve prior loss, parents do suffer various troubles when a healthy child is born, influencing that healthy baby too.

6. Turning Adversity into Transformative Growth

This final section explores how the many adversities that parents encounter, when the unexpected happens and life throws you a curveball, can be reshaped into a positive: whether it's personal growth, becoming an activist, starting a charity, peer support, or other ways that people heal from the experience of adversity. There often is a silver lining in the hardship of healing from complications, or caring for a baby with serious health conditions.

I have found that people who suffer need their concerns to be addressed, and it is why this companion book, also including energy-medicine techniques, has been written to give a voice to those experiences. Their postnatal period does not look at all like the rest of this book, and they could feel excluded from lots of the positive messages that I've been giving throughout *Life After Birth: A Parent's Holistic Guide to Thriving in the Fourth Trimester*. I hope that I have done justice to the reality that they face/have faced. When it comes to perinatal mood and anxiety disorders, it feels so important to describe the real-life experience of mothers and fathers because they are burdened by the impact of stigma.

Stigma is the force that stops mothers and fathers from seeking help. Shining a light on the stigma of mental illness is the first step in eliminating it. And then those 20% of mothers, and some of their partners, who suffer can feel more able to reach out and get the help that they need to recover from perinatal mental illness. Returning to this Guide, to draw this book to a close, here is a final energy-medicine technique for your relaxing pleasure.

Brazilian Toe Technique

Here is a delicious final protocol from energy medicine called the Brazilian Toe Technique. There are numerous benefits. It is highly soothing for people suffering from aches and pains. It helps with stress reduction, insomnia, calming the nervous system, stabilizing emotional imbalances, deep relaxation, and for eliminating the side effects of chemotherapy treatment. It has a positive neurological impact by stimulating the acupuncture points in the toes and feet, and this will calm the brain when it's on "overwhelm."

The technique is an excellent resource for those who are struggling with mental or emotional imbalances. It also helps to move and clear toxins, and grounds the receiver. I can't think of a better way to finish this book than the very yummy experience of being blissed out by the Brazilian Toe Technique.

If I were doing this as a practitioner, there would be preliminary steps to take, but you just need to have some water nearby for a drink, to wash away those toxins that are being cleared. The receiver lays face up, and the giver sits at the feet in a position that allows the giver to remain comfortable. Here's a little table that tells you which toes, and the order to go in, starting with the middle toes and fingers:

Toe #	Thumb and Finger #	
3 Middle toe	Thumb	3 Middle finger
4 Fourth toe	Thumb	4 Ring finger
5 Little toe	Thumb	5 Little finger
2 Index toe	Thumb	2 Index finger
1 Big toe	Thumb	2 & 3 One finger on each corner

You want to hold the toes very lightly, on both feet at the same time in the sequence in the table. Your thumb goes under the pad of the toe, and the other finger rests on the nail of the toe. You want to maintain contact with the foot when you change toes, gently sliding your thumb across to the next toe and then moving the finger on to the nail.

Starting with the middle toe, #3, you hold the toes of both feet for **three minutes** before changing toes. Continue with all the toes for three minutes, and when you get to the big toe, both fingers 2 and 3 will hold each side at the base of the nail. It's that simple. And it will do wonders for your relationship to be sharing a process with each other that will help you feel calm and restored. It might be that the mother gets a number of treatments before she's able to reciprocate, but it's worth it. It's very healing, and it establishes that duet of teamwork that we've talked about in Part 5. Also, it expresses the essence of simplicity that we've been focused on throughout this book on the fourth trimester

As this book draws to its conclusion (and what better way to do that than the Brazilian Toe Technique), I sincerely hope that it helps you get off to the right start. If you have had a difficult transition and suffer from mental health or other baby-related issues, I urge you to read *The Adverse Aftermath of Birth*, which will be published shortly after this one.

Blessed be.

References

Abrams, D.C. (2002). Father nature: The making of a modern dad. *Psychology Today, 35*(2), 38-47.

ACOG Committee on Obstetric Practice. (2018). ACOG committee opinion #736: Optimizing postpartum care: Presidential task force on redefining the postpartum visit. *Obstetrics and Gynecology, 131*(5), e140-e150.

Ainsworth, M. D. S., & Bell, S. M. (1970). Attachment, exploration, and separation: Illustrated by the behavior of one-year-olds in a strange situation. *Child Development, 41,* 49-67.

Amelie.fr. (2017a). *Paternity and childcare leave.* Retrieved from https://www.ameli.fr/assure/droits-demarches/famille/maternite-paternite-adoption/conge-paternite-accueil-enfant.

Amelie.fr. (2017b). *Maternity leave: Duration.* Retrieved from https://www.ameli.fr/assure/droits-demarches/famille/maternite-paternite-adoption/conge-maternite.

American College of Nurse-Midwives. (2016). *CNM/CM birth statistics.* Retrieved from http://www.midwife.org/CNM/CM-attended-Birth-Statistics.

Attachment Parenting International. (2008). *Our mission.* Retrieved from AttachmentParenting.org.

Australian Department of Human Services. (2017). *Day and partner pay.* Retrieved from https://www.humanservices.gov.au/individuals/services/centrelink/dad-and-partner-pay.

Australian Government Fair Work Ombudsman. (n.d.). *Maternity and parental leave.* Retrieved from https://www.fairwork.gov.au/leave/maternity-and-parental-leave.

Australian Government Fair Work Ombudsman. (n.d.). *Taking parental leave.* Retrieved from https://www.fairwork.gov.au/leave/maternity-and-parental-leave/taking-parental-leave.

Axness, M. (2012). *Parenting for peace: Raising the next generation of peacemakers.* Boulder, CO: Sentient Publications. http://marcyaxness.com/book/

Bankhead, C. (2013). *Induced labor linked to higher autism rate. Medpage Today.* Retrieved from http://www.medpagetoday.com/Neurology/Autism/40952.

Barron, D. (2017). The neuroscience of paid parental leave. *Scientific American*. Retrieved from https://blogs.scientificamerican.com/observations/the-neuroscience-of-paid-parentalleave/?utm_source=newsletter&utm_medium=email&utm_campaign=policy&utm_content=link&utm_term=2017-10-30_more-stories.

Beck, C. T., & Watson, S. (2008). Impact of birth trauma on breast-feeding: A tale of two pathways. *Nursing Research, 57*(4), 228-236.

Behnke, A. (2003). The physical and emotional effects of postpartum hormone levels. *International Journal of Childbirth Education, 18*(2), 11-14.

Berens, P., Eglash, A., Malloy, M., Steube, A.M., & the Academy of Breastfeeding Medicine. (2016). ABM clinical protocol #26: Persistent pain with breastfeeding. *Breastfeeding Medicine, 11*(2), 46-53.

Bing, E., & Colman, L. (1977). *Making love during pregnancy*. New York: Bantam Books.

Bolen, J. S. (1985). *Goddesses in everywoman: A new psychology of women*. New York: Harper Colophon Books.

Bowlby, J. (1952). *Maternal care and mental health*. Geneva: World Health Organization.

Bowlby, J. (1969). *Attachment and loss. Vol. 1: Attachment*. New York: Basic Books.

Bowlby, J. (1973). *Attachment and loss. Vol. 2: Separation: Anxiety and anger*. New York: Basic Books.

Bowlby, J. (1980). *Attachment and loss. Vol. 3: Loss: Sadness and depression*, New York: Basic Books.

Boyda-Vikander, S. (2012). *Mothering the mother: 40 days of rest*. Retrieved from http://birthwithoutfearblog.com/2012/10/21/mothering-the-mother-40-days-of-rest/

Brown, A. (2016). *Breastfeeding uncovered: Who really decides how we feed our babies?* London: Pinter & Martin.

Brown University. (2013). MRI study: Breastfeeding boosts babies' brain growth. *Science Daily*. Retrieved from http://www.sciencedaily.com/releases/2013/06/130606141048.htm

Brownmiller, S. (1983). *Femininity*. New York: Linden Press/Simon & Schuster.

Buckley, S.J. (2002). Ecstatic birth: The hormonal blueprint of labor. *Mothering Magazine, 111*, 1-11.

Buckley, S.J. (2009). *Gentle birth, gentle mothering: A doctor's guide to natural childbirth and gentle early parenting choices*, Berkeley, CA: Celestial Arts.

Buckley, S. J. (2015). *Hormonal physiology of childbearing: Evidence and implications for women, babies, and maternity care.* Washington, DC: Childbirth Connection. Retrieved from www.ChildbirthConnection.org/HormonalPhysiology.

Café Mom. (2013). *Are ultrasounds causing autism in unborn babies?* Retrieved from http://www.cafemom.com/group/115890/forums/read/18768280/Are_Ultrasounds_C ausing_Autism_in_Unborn_Babies.

California Work and Family Coalition. (2012). *Six key laws for parents.* Retrieved from http://paidfamilyleave.org/pdf/KeyLawPoster_ENG.pdf.

Callander, M.G., with Travis, J.W. (2012). *Why dads leave: Insights and resources for when partners become parents.* Asheville, NC: Akasha Publications.

Campbell, S.M. (1980). *The couple's journey: Intimacy as a path to wholeness.* San Luis Obispo, CA: Impact Publishers.

Carman, E., & Carman, N. (2013). *Cosmic cradle: Spiritual dimensions of life before birth.* Berkely, CA: North Atlantic Books.

Chamberlain, D.B. (1988). *Babies remember birth: And other extraordinary scientific discoveries about the mind and personality of your newborn.* Los Angeles: Jeremy P. Tarcher, Inc.

Chamberlain, D.B. (1998). *The mind of your newborn baby.* Berkeley, CA: North Atlantic Books.

Chamberlain, D. B. (2013). *Windows to the womb: Revealing the conscious baby from conception to birth.* Berkeley, CA: North Atlantic Books.

Cleiss. (2016). *The French social security system: 1 – Health, maternity, paternity, disability, and death branch; health, maternity and paternity insurance.* Retrieved from http://www.cleiss.fr/docs/regimes/regime_france/an_1.html.

Colson, S.D. (2010). *An introduction to biological nurturing: New angles on breastfeeding.* Amarillo, TX: Praeclarus Press.

Condon, J.C., Jeyasuria, P., Faust, J.M., & Mendelson, J.R. (2004). Surfactant protein secreted by the maturing mouse fetal lung acts as a hormone that signals the initiation of parturition. *PNAS, 101*(14), 4978-4983. https://doi.org/10.1073/pnas.0401124101

Craig, G. (n.d). How to do the EFT tapping basics - The basic recipe. *The Gary Craig Official EFT Training Centers.* Retrieved from https://www.emofree.com/eft-tutorial/tapping- basics/how-to-do-eft.html.

Crockford, C., Deschner, T., Zieglar, T.E., & Wittig, R.M. (2014). Endogenous peripheral oxytocin measures can give insight into the dynamics of social relationships: A review. *Frontiers in Behavioral Neuroscience, 8,* Article 68; doi: 10.3389/fnbeh.2014.00068.

Daub, C. (2007). *Birthing in the spirit.* Medford, NJ: Birth Works Press.

Davies, R. (2012). *Let's put Facebook's 'no nipples' rule to test with your breastfeeding photos.* Retrieved from https://www.theguardian.com/commentisfree/2012/feb/22/facebook-no-nipples-rule-breastfeeding

Dekker, R. (2017). The evidence on placenta encapsulation. *Evidence-based birth.* Retrieved from https://evidencebasedbirth.com/evidence-on-placenta-encapsulation/.

DelliQuadri, L., & Breckenridge, K. (1978). *Mother care: Helping yourself through the emotional and physical transitions of new motherhood.* New York: Pocket Books.

Dowling, C. (1981).*The Cinderella complex: Women's hidden fear of independence.* New York: Summit Books.

Doyle, K. (n.d.). Out of hospital births on the rise in U.S. *Scientific American.* Retrieved from https://www.scientificamerican.com/article/out-of-hospital-births-on-the-rise-in-u-s/.

Duke University Medical Center. (2012). Newly discovered breast milk antibodies help neutralize HIV. *Science Daily.* Retrieved from http://www.sciencedaily.com/releases/2012/05/120522152653.htm.

Eden, D. (2015). *Donna Eden's daily energy routine* [OFFICIAL VERSION]. Retrieved from https://www.youtube.com/watch?v=Di5Ua44iuXc.

Eden, D., & Feinstein, D. (1998). *Energy medicine.* New York: Jeremy P. Tarcher/Putnam.

Eden, D., & Feinstein, D. (2009). *Energy medicine for women: Aligning your body's energies to boost your health and vitality.* London: Piatkus.

Eden, D., & Feinstein, D. (2012a). Class 2 Handout. *Eden Energy Medicine Certification Program:* Ashland, OR: Innersource.

Eden, D., & Feinstein, D. (2012b). Class 4 Handout. *Eden Energy Medicine Certification Program:* Ashland, OR: Innersource.

Eden, D., & Feinstein, D. (2004-2011). *Energies of love: The invisible key to a fulfilling relationship* DVD. Retrieved from www.innersource.net.

Eden, D., & Feinstein, D. (2014). *The energies of love: Using energy medicine to keep your relationship thriving.* London: Piatkus.

Elding, C. (2013). Formula vs. breastfeeding. *Health Cloud.* Retrieved from https://www.thehealthcloud.co.uk/formula-vs-breastfeeding/.

England, D.C. (2017). *Lactation accommodation: Mandatory breaks for breastfeeding in California.* Retrieved from https://www.nolo.com/legal-encyclopedia/lactation-accommodation-mandatory-breaks-breastfeeding-california.html

England, D.C. (n.d.). *Pregnancy discrimination: When you should talk to a lawyer.* Retrieved from https://www.nolo.com/legal-encyclopedia/pregnancy-discrimination-when-you-should-talk-lawyer.html.

Entrepreneur. (2017). *19 Companies and industries with radically awesome parental leave policies. Entrepreneur*: Retrieved from https://www.entrepreneur.com/slideshow/249467.

Entrust. (2017). *Baby's first crawl – Initiation of breastfeeding.* Retrieved from https://www.youtube.com/watch?v=0KVAOUILFq0.

Equinet (European Network of Equality Bodies). (2014). *France – Discrimination against pregnant workers.* Retrieved from http://www.equineteurope.org/DescriptionAn-awareness-raising.

Erickson, E.N., & Emeis, C. (2017). Breastfeeding outcomes after oxytocin use during childbirth: An integrative review. *Journal of Midwifery & Women's Health, 62*(4), 397-417, doi:10.1111/jmwh.12601.

Expatica. (2016). *Having a baby in France and maternity leave in France.* Retrieved from https://www.expatica.com/fr/healthcare/Having-a-baby-in-France_107664.html.

Fairgodboss. (2017). *Pregnancy, maternity leave, and paternity leave in Washington State.* Retrieved from https://fairygodboss.com/career-topics/pregnancy-maternity-leave-and-paternity-leave-in-washington-state.

Fairygodboss. (n.d.). *Pregnancy and maternity leave for New Jersey employees.* Retrieved from https://fairygodboss.com/career-topics/pregnancy-and-maternity-leave-for-new-jersey-employees.

Feldman, R. (2012). Oxytocin and social affiliation in humans. *Hormones and Behavior, 61,* 380-391.

Ford, G. (2006). *The (new) contented little baby book.* London: Vermillion.

French Mamma. (n.d.). *Maternity leave in France.* Retrieved from http://frenchmamma.com/maternity-leave-france/.

Galvao, D.M.P.G., & Silva, I.A. (2013). The approach to breastfeeding in the first years of elementary school. *Rev Esc Enferm USP, 47*(2), 468-476.

Gao, L. Rabbitt, E.H., Condon, J.C., Renthal, N.E., Johnston, J.M., Mitsche, M.A., Chambon, P., Xu, J., O'Malley, B.W., & Mendelson, C.R. (2015). Steroid receptor coactivators 1 and 2 mediate fetal-to-maternal signaling that initiates parturition. *Journal of Clinical Investigation, 125*(7), 2808-2824

Gaskin, I.M. (2009). *Ina May's guide to breastfeeding.* New York: Bantam Books.

Ginott, H. (1965/2010). *Between parent and child: New solutions to old problems.* New York: Avon Books.

Gottman, J.M., & Gottman, J.S. (2007). *And baby makes three: The six-step plan for preserving marital intimacy and rekindling romance after baby arrives.* New York: Three Rivers Press.

Gottman, J.M., & Silver, N. (1999). *The 7 principles for making marriage work.* New York: Three Rivers Press.

Gov.UK. (n.d.). *Maternity pay and leave.* Retrieved from https://www.gov.uk/maternity-pay-leave.

Gov.UK. (n.d.). *Shared parental leave and pay.* Retrieved from https://www.gov.uk/shared- parental-leave-and-pay.

Hamil, D. (2011). Brain growth linked to duration of pregnancy and how long babies suckle. *Medical News Today.* Retrieved from http://www.medicalnewstoday.com/releases/220481.php.

Harman, T., & Wakeford, A. (2014). Microbirth. *Alto Films.* Retrieved from http://microbirth.com/the-film/.

Harris, P. (2017). *The daily energy routine.* Retrieved from https://youtu.be/nN2uq78Y2bE.

Harries, V., & Brown, A. (2017). The association between use of infant parenting books that promote strict routines, and maternal depression, self-efficacy, and parenting confidence. *Early Child Development and Care,* doi:10.108 0/03004430.2017.1378650. Retrieved from https://www.tandfonline.com/doi/full/10.1080/03004430.2017.1378650

Hartley, M., & Commire, A. (1990). *Breaking the silence.* New York: G.P. Putnam's Sons.

HeartMath Institute. *Quick coherence˚ technique.* Retrieved from https://www.heartmath.com/quick-coherence-technique/.

Hendricks, G., & Hendricks, K. (1990). *Conscious loving: The journey to co-commitment.* New York: Bantam Books.

Heslett, C., Hedberg, S., & Rumble, H. (2007). *Did you ever wonder what's in…?* New Westminster, BC, Canada: Breastfeeding Course for Health Care Providers, Douglas College.

House of Commons Women and Equalities Select Committee. (2016). *Pregnancy and maternity discrimination: First report of session 2016-2017.* Retrieved from https://publications.parliament.uk/pa/cm201617/cmselect/cmwomeq/90/90.pdf.

Hurst, N.M. (2007). Recognizing and treating delayed or failed lactogenesis II. *Journal of Midwifery & Women's Health, 52*(6), 588-594. Retrieved from https://www.medscape.com/viewarticle/565620_2.

Instant Offices. (2017). *Maternity leave around the world.* Retrieved from http://www.instantoffices.com/blog/featured/maternity-leave-around-world/.

Institute of HeartMath. (n.d.). The power of emotion. *E-booklet by HeartMath Institute.* Retrieved from www.hearthmath.org.

Johnson, S. (2011). *Hold me tight: Your guide to the most successful approach to building loving relationships.* London: Piatkus.

Johnson, S. (2011). *Integrating heart and soul: The new science of attachment & EFT.* Retrieved from https://youtu.be/3bgod5TRgrI.

Jones, G.L., Morrell, C.J., Cooke, J.M., Speier, D., Anumba, D., & Stewart-Brown, S. (2011). The development of two postnatal health instruments: One for mothers (M-PHI) and one for fathers (F-PHI) to measure health during the first year of parenting. *Quality of Life Research, 20*(7), 1011–1022.

Jones, W. (2017). *The importance of dads and grandmas to the breastfeeding mother.* Amarillo, TX: Praeclarus Press.

Keen, S. (1983). *The passionate life: Stages of loving.* San Francisco: Harper & Row, Publishers.

Kemp, R. (2016). Why are only 1 in 100 men taking up shared parental leave? *The Telegraph.* Retrieved from http://www.telegraph.co.uk/men/the-filter/why-are-only-1-in-100-men-taking-up-shared-parental-leave/.

Kendall-Tackett, K. (2007). A new paradigm for depression in new mothers: The central role of inflammation and how breastfeeding and anti-inflammatory treatments protect maternal mental health. *International Breastfeeding Journal, 2*(6), doi: 10.1186/1746-4358-2-6.

Kendall-Tackett, K., Cong, Z., & Hale, T.W. (2015). Birth interventions related to lower rates of exclusive breastfeeding and increased risks of postpartum depression in a large sample. *Clinical Lactation, 6*(3). Retrieved from http://dx.doi.org/10.1891/2158-0782.6.3.87

Kendall-Tackett, K.A. (2009). Psychological trauma and physical health: A psychoneuroimmunology approach to etiology of negative health effects and possible interventions. *Psychological Trauma, 1,* 35-48.

Kendall-Tackett, K.A., Cong, Z., & Hale, T.W. (2011). The effect of feeding method on sleep duration, maternal well-being, and postpartum depression. *Clinical Lactation, 2*(2), 22-26.

Klaus, M.H., & Kennell, J.H. (1976). *Maternal-infant bonding.* St. Louis, MO: C.V. Mosby Company.

Klaus, M.H., Kennell, J.H., & Klaus, P.H. (1996). *Bonding: Building the foundations of secure attachment and independence,* Revised Edition. Boston: Da Capo Press.

Klaus, M.H., & Klaus, P. (1998). *Your amazing newborn.* Cambridge, MA: Da Capo Press.

Kramer, J. (2012). The woman on the cover is both Madonna and whore. *Kindred Media.* Retrieved from http://kindredmedia.org/2012/05/the-woman-on-the-cover-is-both-madonna-and-whore/.

La Leche League International. (1976). *The womanly art of breastfeeding.* Franklin Park, IL: La Leche League International.

Lawlor, M. (2012). *U.S. midwifery organizations make the case for normal physiologic birth.* NACPM press release.

Lawyers Alliance. (2009). *Legal Alert: Right of Nursing Mothers to Express Breast Milk Summary.* Retrieved from http://www.lawyersalliance.org/pdfs/news_legal/June_09_Alert_Right_of_Nursing_Mothers_to_Express.pdf.

Legal Aid at Work. (n.d.). *Work and family.* Retrieved from https://legalaidatwork.org/our-programs/work-and-family-program/.

LeMasters, E. E. (1957). Parenthood as crisis. *Marriage and Family Living, 19,* 352-355.

Lozada, Adriana. (2015). *Life with a newborn: Why it's so hard to take a shower* video. Retrieved from https://www.youtube.com/watch?v=oQt90SHj6iY&feature=youtu.be.

Maternity Action. (n.d.). *Shared parental leave and pay.* Retrieved from https://www.maternityaction.org.uk/advice-2/mums-dads-scenarios/shared-parental -leave-and-pay/.

Maternity Action. (2017). *End unfair redundancies,#maternityrights.* Retrieved from https://www.maternityactioncampaigns.org.uk/wpcontent/uploads/2017/11/Redunda ncyReportFinal.compressed.pdf

Matthews, V. (2008). *The relationship puzzle: The five element way to harmonize interactions DVD.* Retrieved from www.vickimatthrews.com.

McCarty, W.A. (2012). *Welcoming consciousness: Supporting babies' wholeness from the beginning of life.* Santa Barbara, CA: Wondrous Beginnings Publishing.

McCraty, R., & Childre, D. (2002). The appreciative heart: The psychophysiology of postive emotions and optimal functioning. Boulder Creek, CA *HeartMath Research Center, Institute of HealthMath*, Publication No. 02-026.

McCraty, Rollin. (2006). Emotional stress, positive emotions and psychophysiological coherence. In B. Bengt & R.E. Arnetz (Eds.). *Stress in health and disease* (pp. 342-365). Weinheim, Germany: Wiley-VCH.

McCraty, R. (2015). *Science of the heart: Exploring the role of the heart in human performance, vol.2*, Boulder Creek, CA: HeartMath Research Center, HeartMath Institute.

Meinlschmidt, G., Martin, C., Neumann, I.D., & Heinrichs, M. (2010). Maternal cortisol in late pregnancy and hypothalamic-pituitary-adrenal reactivity to psychosocial stress postpartum in women. *Stress, 13*(2), 163–171.

Mendelsohn, R. S. (1984). *How to raise a healthy child...in spite of your doctor.* Chicago, IL: Contemporary Books Inc.

Mohrbacher, N. (2013). *Breastfeeding solutions: Quick tips for the most common nursing challenges,* Oakland, CA: New Harbinger Publications.

Mohrbacher, N., & Kendall-Tackett, K. (2010). *Breastfeeding made simple,* 2nd Edition, Oakland, CA: New Harbinger Publications.

Moore, E.R., Bergman, N., Anderson, G.C., & Medley, N. (2016). Early skin-to-skin contact for mothers and their healthy newborn infants. *Cochrane Database of Systematic Reviews, 11.* Art. No.: CD003519. DOI: 10.1002/14651858.CD003519.pub4.

Morton, J. (2016). *5 tips to help you express breast milk easily.* Retrieved from https://www.youtube.com/watch?v=EFSqetb9u9Y&feature=youtu.be.

National Partnership for Women and Families. (2017). *State paid family leave insurance laws.* Retrieved from http://www.nationalpartnership.org/research-library/work -family/paid-leave/state-paid-family-leave-laws.pdf.

National Conference of State Legislatures. (2016). *State family and medical leave laws.* Retrieved from http://www.ncsl.org/research/labor-and-employment/state-family-and-medical-leave-laws.aspx.

New York State Labor Law. (2009). *Guidelines regarding the rights of nursing mothers to express milk in the work place.* Retrieved from https://www.labor.ny.gov/workerprotection/laborstandards/pdfs/guidelinesexpressionofbreastmilkfinal.pdf.

Newman, J. (2011). *Asymmetrical latch.* Retrieved from https://www.youtube.com/watch?v=NO5ZDKynaD0&feature=youtu.be.

Newton, N. (1963/1955). *Maternal emotions*. New York: Paul B Hoeber.

Nierop, A., Bratsikas, A., Zimmermann, R., & Ehlert, U. (2006). Are stress-induced cortisol changes during pregnancy associated with postpartum depressive symptoms? *Psychosomatic Medicine, 68*, 931–937.

Nichols, J. (2010). Healthy birth practice #1: Let labor begin on its own. *Science & Sensibility*. Retrieved from https://www.scienceandsensibility.org/p/bl/et/blogid=2&blogaid=232.

O'Neill, N., & O'Neill, G. (1972). *Open marriage: A new life style for couples*. New York: Avon Books.

Peaceful Parenting. (2008). *Fetal lungs protein release triggers labor to begin*. Retrieved from http://www.drmomma.org/2008/01/fetal-lungs-protein-release-triggers.html.

Pearce, J.C. (1977). *The magical child*. New York: Bantam Books (reissued in 1992 by Plume).

Pickert, K. (2012). The man who remade motherhood. *Time Magazine*. Retrieved from http://time.com/606/the-man-who-remade-motherhood/

Polettini, J., Behnia, F., Taylor, B.D., Saade, G.R., Taylor, R.N., & Menon, R. (2015). Telomere fragment induced amnion cell senescence: A contributor to parturition? *PLOS ONE, 10*(9), e0137188 DOI: 10.1371/journal.pone.0137188

Porter, L.L. (2009). *The science of attachment: Biological roots of love*. Retrieved from http://www.naturalchild.org/guest/lauren_lindsey_porter.html.

Pryor, K. (1977). *Nursing your baby,* Revised Edition, New York: Pocket Books.

Raphael, D. (1976). *The tender gift: Breastfeeding. Mothering the mother – the way to successful breastfeeding*. New York: Schocken Books.

Rodgers, C. (2006). Questions about prenatal ultrasound and the alarming increase in autism. *Midwifery Today, 80*. Retrieved from http://www.midwiferytoday.com/articles/ultrasoundrodgers.asp.

Sabel, V. (2012). *The Blossom Method™: The revolutionary way to communicate with your baby from birth*. London: Vermilion.

Salzberg, S. (1995). *Lovingkindness: The revolutionary art of happiness*. Boston: Shambala Publications Inc.

Sears, M., & Sears, W. (2000). *The breastfeeding book: Everything you need to know about nursing your child from birth through weaning,* New York: Little, Brown & Co.

Sears, W., & Sears, M. (2001). *The attachment parenting book:
A commonsense guide to understanding and nurturing your baby.*
New York: Little, Brown and Co.

Siegel, D. (2010). *Mindsight: Transform your brain with the new science of
kindness.* Oxford, England: Oneworld Publications.

Siegel, D. (2011). *How mindfulness can change the wiring of our brains.*
NICABM webinar series. Retrieved from https://www.nicabm.com/
mindfulness-seeing-the-impact-of-mindfulness-in-the-brain/

Siegel, D. (2013). Post on Facebook, June 3, 2013.

Speier, D.S. (2001). Becoming a mother. *Journal of the Association for Research
on Mothering, 3*(1) 7-18.

Speier, D.S. (2002). *The childbirth educator as ethnographer: A feminist
retrospective ethnography of a professional practice.* Unpublished PhD
thesis, University of Manchester.

Speier, D.S. (2017). Birth trauma. In P. Leach (Ed.). *Transforming infant
wellbeing: Research, policy and practice for the first 1001 critical days*
(pp. 107-116). London: Routledge.

Stephenson, J. (2016). Only half of babies in England now delivered by
midwives. *Nursing Times.* Retrieved from https://www.nursingtimes.
net/news/hospital/only-half-of-babies-in-england-now-delivered-by-
midwives/7013310.article.

Supporting Healthy and Normal Physiologic Childbirth:
A Consensus Statement by ACNM, MANA, and NACPM. (2013).
The Journal of Perinatal Education, 22(1), 14–18. Retrieved from
http://doi.org/10.1891/1058-1243.22.1.14.

Supporting Working Parents. (2015a). Returning to work from leave:
What role am I entitled to when I return to work. *Australian
Government Initiative.* Retrieved from https://supportingworkingparents.
humanrights.gov.au/employees/returning-work
-leave#what-role-am-i-entitled-to-when-i-return-to-work.

Supporting Working Parents. (2015b). Returning to work from leave:
Do I have any rights if I breastfeed/express in the work place. *Australian
Government Initiative.* Retrieved from https://supportingworkingparents.
humanrights.gov.au/employees/returning-work-leave#do-i-have-any-
rights-if-i-breastfeedexpress-in-the-workplace.

Tannen, D. (1990). *You just don't understand: Women and men in conversation.*
New York: Ballantine Books.

Taylor, E. (2014). *Becoming us: 8 steps to grow a family that thrives.* Sydney, Australia: Three Turtles Press.

The Bub Hub Crew. (2017). A guide to parental leave pay in Australia – are you eligible? *The Bub Hub.* Retrieved from https://www.bubhub.com.au/hubbub-blog/paid-parental-leave-pay-australia/.

Ultrasound-Autism.org. (n.d.). *Ultrasound autism connection.* Retrieved from http://www.ultrasound-autism.org/.

U.S. Department of Labor. (n.d.). *State-level workplace breastfeeding rights.* Retrieved from https://www.dol.gov/wb/maps/4.htm.

U.S. Department of Labor, Wage and Hour Division. (n.d.a). *Break time for nursing mothers.* Retrieved from https://www.dol.gov/whd/nursingmothers/.

U.S. Department of Labor, Wage and Hour Division. (n.d.b). *Section 7(r) of the fair labor standards act, break time for nursing mothers provision.* Retrieved from https://www.dol.gov/whd/nursingmothers/Sec7rFLSA_btnm.htm.

UT Southwestern Medical Center. (2015). Molecular mechanisms within fetal lungs initiate labor [*Science Daily*]. Retrieved from http://www.sciencedaily.com/releases/2015/06/150622162023.htm.

University of Texas Medical Branch at Galveston. (2015). Scientists uncover signal for when a pregnant woman is about to go into labor [*Science Daily*]. Retrieved from http://www.sciencedaily.com/releases/2015/10/151026132136.htm?utm_source=fee dburner&utm_medium=email&utm_campaign=Feed%3A+sciencedaily%2Fhealth_medicine%2Fpregnancy_and_childbirth+%28Pregnancy+and+Childbirth+News+--+ScienceDaily%29.

Uvnas Moberg, K. (2011/2003). *The oxytocin factor: Tapping the hormone of calm, love, and healing.* London: Pinter and Martin Ltd.

Verny, T., with Kelly, J. (1981). *The secret life of the unborn child.* New York: Summit Books.

Watson, J.B. (1928). *Psychological care of infant and child.* New York: W.W. Norton & Co.

White, C. (2010). *The forms of attachment.* Retrieved from http://www.essentialparenting.com/2010/05/22/the-forms-of-attachment/.

Wildner, K. (2012). Kangaroo care. *Midwifery Today, 101.* Retrieved from https://midwiferytoday.com/mt-articles/kangaroo-care/.

Winder, K. (n.d., updated 5/2/17). *Lactation cookies – 90% of our fans say this recipe works!* Retrieved from https://www.bellybelly.com.au/breastfeeding/lactation-cookies/#.Ui8IlMZwqa8

Woo, M. (2017). *This maternity leave registry site lets you crowdfund time with your baby* [*Offspring*]. Retrieved from https://offspring.lifehacker.com/this-maternity-leave-registry-site-lets-you-crowdfund-t-1818502196.

World Economic Forum. (2016). *Rankings: Global gender gap index 2016.* Retrieved from http://reports.weforum.org/global-gender-gap-report-2016/rankings/.

Zanardo, V., Nicolussi, S., Carlo, G., Marzari, F., Faggiano, D., Favaro, F., & Plebani, M. (2001). Beta endorphin concentrations in human milk. *Journal of Pediatric Gastroenterology & Nutrition, 33*(2), 160-164.

Resources

Baby Center websites: www.babycenter.com or www.babycentre.co.uk.

Baby Gooroo. (n.d.). https://babygooroo.com/articles/10-benefits-of-skin-to-skin-contact.

Barston, S. *Fearless formula feeder: Standing up for formula feeders without being a boob about it.* Retrieved from http://www.fearlessformulafeeder.com/.

Meehan, K. *Birth healing.* Retrieved from http://www.birthhealing.com.

Digital Doula® App, a companion postpartum application that accompanies this book with additional information and resources, available in iOS and Android. Retrieved from http://digitaldoula.com/.

To learn more about Donna Eden and Eden Energy Medicine go to: www.LearnEnergyMedicine.com.

CPSIA information can be obtained
at www.ICGtesting.com
Printed in the USA
FSHW011942281019
63509FS